Diagnostic Imaging of the Teeth and Jaws

Editor

GALAL OMAMI

DENTAL CLINICS OF NORTH AMERICA

www.dental.theclinics.com

April 2024 • Volume 68 • Number 2

ELSEVIER

1600 John F. Kennedy Boulevard ● Suite 1800 ● Philadelphia, Pennsylvania, 19103-2899

http://www.dental.theclinics.com

DENTAL CLINICS OF NORTH AMERICA Volume 68, Number 2
April 2024 ISSN 0011-8532, ISBN: 978-0-443-12139-5

Editor: John Vassallo; j.vassallo@elsevier.com
Developmental Editor: Akshay Samson

Dental Clinics of North America (ISSN 0011-8532) is published quarterly by Elsevier Inc., 360 Park Avenue South, New York, NY 10010-1710. Months of issue are January, April, July, and October. Business and Editorial Offices: 1600 John F. Kennedy Boulevard, Suite 1800, Philadelphia, PA 19103-2899. Periodicals postage paid at New York, NY and additional mailing offices. Subscription prices are $333.00 per year (domestic individuals), $100.00 per year (domestic students/residents), $396.00 per year (Canadian individuals), $100.00 per year (Canadian students/residents) $463.00 per year (international individuals), and $200.00 per year (international students/residents). For institutional access pricing please contact Customer Service via the contact information below. International air speed delivery is included in all *Clinics* subscription prices. All prices are subject to change without notice. **POSTMASTER:** Send address changes to *Dental Clinics of North America*, Elsevier Health Sciences Division, Subscription Customer Service, 3251 Riverport Lane, Maryland Heights, MO 63043. **Customer Service (orders, claims, online, change of address): Elsevier Health Sciences Division, Subscription Customer Service, 3251 Riverport Lane, Maryland Heights, MO 63043. Tel: 1-800-654-2452 (U.S. and Canada). Fax: 314-447-8029. E-mail: journalscustomerservice-usa@elsevier.com (for print support); journalsonlinesupport-usa@elsevier.com (for online support).**

Reprints. For copies of 100 or more, of articles in this publication, please contact the Commercial Reprints Department, Elsevier Inc., 360 Park Avenue South, New York, NY 10010-1710. Tel.: 212-633-3874; Fax: 212-633-3820; E-mail: reprints@elsevier.com.

The Dental Clinics of North America is covered in *MEDLINE/PubMed (Index Medicus), Current Contents/Clinical Medicine, ISI/BIOMED* and *Cinahl.*

Contributors

EDITOR

GALAL OMAMI, BDS, MSc, MDentSc, FRCD(C)
Diplomate, American Board of Oral and Maxillofacial Radiology, Associate Professor, Division of Oral Diagnosis, Oral Medicine, and Oral Radiology, Department of Oral Health Practice, University of Kentucky College of Dentistry, Lexington, Kentucky

AUTHORS

SARAH E. AGUIRRE, DDS, MS, DABOMP
Assistant Professor, Department of Diagnostic Sciences, College of Dentistry, The University of Tennessee Health Science Center, Memphis, Tennessee

FIRAS AL YAFI, DDS, MS
Diplomate of the American Board of Periodontology; Diplomate, Arab Board of Oral Surgery, Periodontist, Private Practice, Plano, Texas

ABEER ALHADIDI, DDS, MS, PhD
Diplomate, American Board of Oral and Maxillofacial Radiology, Clinical Associate Professor of Oral and Maxillofacial Radiology, Oral and Maxillofacial Pathology, Radiology, and Medicine, NYU College of Dentistry, New York, New York; School of Dentistry, The University of Jordan, Amman, Jordan

NOURA ALSUFYANI, BDS, MSc, PhD, DIPFHID
Associate Professor, Department of Oral Medicine and Diagnostic Sciences, Oral and Maxillofacial Radiology, College of Dentistry, King Saud University, Riyadh, Saudi Arabia; Department of Medicine and Dentistry, Adjunct Professor, Department of Medicine and Dentistry, University of Alberta, Canada

ADEL ALZAHRANI, BDS, MDS
Assistant Professor, Department of Oral Medicine and Diagnostic Sciences, Oral and Maxillofacial Radiology, College of Dentistry, King Saud University, Riyadh, Saudi Arabia

BARTON F. BRANSTETTER IV, MD
Professor, Department of Radiology, University of Pittsburgh Medical Center, Pittsburgh, Pennsylvania

ARISTIDES A. CAPIZZANO, MD
Clinical Associate Professor, Division of Neuroradiology, University of Michigan, Ann Arbor, Michigan

ADEYINKA F. DAYO, BDS, MS
Assistant Professor, Department of Oral Medicine, School of Dental Medicine, University of Pennsylvania, Philadelphia, Pennsylvania

YAZAN HASSONA, BDS, MFDSRCSI, FFDRCSI (OSOM), PhD
Professor of Oral Medicine and Special Care Dentistry, School of Dentistry, The University of Jordan, Dean, School of Dentistry, Al Ahliyya University, Amman, Jordan

ABDO ISMAIL, DDS, MS
Periodontist, Private Practice, Arlington, Texas

PHOEBE PUI YING LAM, BDS, MDS, MPaedDentRCS
Clinical Assistant Professor in Paediatric Dentistry, Faculty of Dentistry, The University of Hong Kong, Prince Philip Dental Hospital, Sai Ying Pun, Hong Kong

CRAIG S. MILLER, DMD, MS
Professor, Division of Oral Diagnosis, Oral Medicine, and Oral Radiology, University of Kentucky College of Dentistry, Lexington, Kentucky

GALAL OMAMI, BDS, MSc, MDentSc, FRCD(C)
Diplomate, American Board of Oral and Maxillofacial Radiology, Associate Professor, Division of Oral Diagnosis, Oral Medicine, and Oral Radiology, Department of Oral Health Practice, University of Kentucky College of Dentistry, Lexington, Kentucky

TEMITOPE T. OMOLEHINWA, BDS, DMD, DScD, DABOM
Assistant Professor, Department of Oral Medicine, School of Dental Medicine, University of Pennsylvania, Philadelphia, Pennsylvania

ADEPITAN A. OWOSHO, DDS, DABOMP, FAAOM
Associate Professor, Department of Diagnostic Sciences, College of Dentistry, The University of Tennessee Health Science Center, Memphis, Tennessee

FRANCISCO RIVAS-RODRIGUEZ, MD
Clinical Associate Professor, Division of Neuroradiology, University of Michigan, Ann Arbor, Michigan

ILSON SEPÚLVEDA A, DDS, MSc
Assistant Professor, Finis Terrae University School of Dentistry, Santiago, Chile; Radiology Department, ENT-Head and Neck Surgery and Maxillofacial Services, General Hospital of Concepción, Concepción, Chile

WERNER H. SHINTAKU, DDS, MS, MS, DABOMR
Professor, Department of Diagnostic Sciences, College of Dentistry, The University of Tennessee Health Science Center, Memphis, Tennessee

ALI Z. SYED, BDS, MHA, MS
Associate Professor, Director of OMR Clinic, Department of Oral and Maxillofacial Medicine and Diagnostic Sciences, Case Western Reserve University School of Dental Medicine, Cleveland, Ohio

RICHARD H. WIGGINS III, MD, CIIP, FSIIM
Professor, Department of Radiology and Imaging Sciences, University of Utah Health Sciences Center, Salt Lake City, Utah

MELVYN YEOH, MD, DMD, FACS
Associate Professor, Division of Oral and Maxillofacial Surgery, University of Kentucky College of Dentistry, Lexington, Kentucky

Contents

DENTAL CLINICS OF NORTH AMERICA

SERIES OF RELATED INTEREST

Atlas of the Oral and Maxillofacial Surgery Clinics
https://www.oralmaxsurgeryatlas.theclinics.com/

Oral and Maxillofacial Surgery Clinics
https://www.oralmaxsurgery.theclinics.com/

Preface

Diagnostic Imaging of the Teeth and Jaws

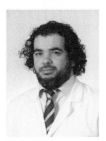

Galal Omami, BDS, MSc, MDentSc,
FRCD(C), Dip. ABOMR
Editor

I am pleased to help bring forth this issue of *Dental Clinics of North America* focusing on assessment and interpretation of oral and maxillofacial radiographic images. The aim of this issue is to provide readers with a comprehensive and up-to-date imaging interpretation of abnormalities related to the dental and maxillofacial complex. This issue includes 11 articles, all of which are designed to be highly practical and focused on assessments directly applicable to clinical practice. The breadth of authors and quality of articles testify to the world-class talent contributing to this issue of *Dental Clinics of North America*.

An attempt has been made to include many common abnormalities that may produce radiographic changes in the jaws and uncommon abnormalities as well, so that the issue can be used as a practical reference. Basic principles of radiographic interpretation have been kept in mind, and an attempt was made to correlate the pathologic changes with those revealed in the radiographic images.

It is not uncommon for the initial evidence of serious local or general disease to be revealed in dental radiographs, and all too often that evidence is either not recognized or not identified, sometimes with dire results to the patient. Awareness of the various abnormalities and their possible radiographic appearances is the best insurance against failing to identify the presence and nature of those abnormalities.

It is my hope that readers will find much to interest them here and may perhaps be stimulated to acquire greater knowledge of this special branch of dentistry. I greatly appreciate the time and expertise of the authors who have contributed to this issue. I am also grateful to the editorial and production staff of Elsevier for their guidance and assistance. Finally, I am especially thankful to my family for the time to devote to this task.

Galal Omami, BDS, MSc, MDentSc, FRCD(C), Dip. ABOMR
Division of Oral Diagnosis,
Oral Medicine, and Oral Radiology
Department of Oral Health Practice
University of Kentucky College of Dentistry
770 Rose Street, MN320
Lexington, KY 40536, USA

E-mail address:
galal.omami@uky.edu

Developmental and Acquired Abnormalities of the Teeth

Abeer AlHadidi, DDS, MS, PhD, DIPLOMATE (ABOMR)[a,b,*],
Phoebe Pui Ying Lam, BDS, MDS, MPaedDentRCS[c],
Yazan Hassona, BDS, MFDSRCSI, FFDRCSI (OSOM), PhD[b,d]

KEYWORDS

- Congenital anomalies of teeth • Caries • Resorptive lesions
- Oral and maxillofacial radiology

KEY POINTS

- Cone-beam computed tomography (CBCT) should not be recommended for caries diagnosis due to several major drawbacks, including scatter artifact from metallic restorations, inferior resolution, radiation dosage, and applicability.
- CBCT is the imaging modality of choice in the characterization and differentiation of external and internal resorptive lesions.
- CBCT plays a role in the diagnosis and management of congenital anomalies of teeth.
- A multidisciplinary approach is crucial for managing congenital anomalies of teeth number, size, form, and structure.

INTRODUCTION

Diagnostic imaging plays a pivotal role in the assessment and management of various dental abnormalities, both developmental and acquired. This article presents a detailed analysis of the most common developmental and acquired dental abnormalities (summerized in **Table 1**) and highlights how diagnostic imaging can aid in the accurate identification and thus management of these conditions.

CARIOUS LESIONS
Definition

Dental caries refers to the demineralization of tooth structure resulting from the acidic metabolites produced by the cariogenic bacteria present in the dental plaque.[1]

[a] Oral and Maxillofacial Pathology, Radiology, and Medicine, NYU College of Dentistry, 345 East 24th Street, New York, NY 10010, USA; [b] School of Dentistry, The University of Jordan, Queen Rania Street, Amman, Jordan 11942; [c] The University of Hong Kong, Prince Philip Dental Hospital, 34 Hospital Road, Sai Ying Pun, Hong Kong; [d] School of Dentistry, Al Ahliyya University
* Corresponding author.
E-mail address: aa11678@nyu.edu

Dent Clin N Am 68 (2024) 227–245
https://doi.org/10.1016/j.cden.2023.09.001
0011-8532/24/© 2023 Elsevier Inc. All rights reserved.

Table 1		
Overview of common aquired and congenital dental anomalies		
Acquired Dental Anomalies		
	Carious lesions Non-carious lesions (attrition, abrasion, erosion, abfraction) Resorptive lesions (external and internal resorption)	
Congenital dental anomalies		
	Congenital anomalies of teeth number	Hypodontia Hyperdontia
	Congenital anomalies of teeth size	Microdontia Macrodontia
	Congenital anomalies of teeth form and structure	Localized processes
		Gemination and fusion Concresence Taurodontism Dens invaginatus Dens evaginatus Dilaceration Enamel pearl Turner's hypoplasia
	Regional and generalized diseases	Hereditary amelogenesis imperfecta Hereditary dentine disorder Dentin dysplasia Regional odontodysplasia

Radiographic examinations facilitate the early detection of caries lesions, which is essential to revert the process with remineralization and preserve healthy tooth structure. Owing to the loss of mineralized tooth structure, dental caries appears radiolucent compared with the normal enamel and dentine.

Imaging Techniques and Findings

Bitewing radiographs are the standard of care for posterior caries detection; however, their sensitivity and specificity fluctuate with the lesion location, depth, and stage, as well as the projection geometry (**Fig. 1**). The bitewing examination may be supplemented by periapical views, depending on the patient's specific needs.

Panoramic imaging is suboptimal for caries diagnosis due to geometric distortion and unequal magnification across the image as well as overlapping of teeth and various artifacts associated with improper patient positioning that negatively affect the image quality. Cone-beam computed tomography (CBCT) imaging should not be recommended as a routine for caries diagnosis due to several major drawbacks, including scatter artifact from metallic restorations, inferior resolution, radiation dosage, and applicability.[2]

Proximal caries

Posterior bitewings remain the gold standard for detecting proximal caries, with a high specificity irrespective of the lesion depth. The shape of proximal caries confined to enamel appears to be triangular, with the base at the enamel outer surface and apex pointing toward the dentinoenamel junction (DEJ). Because the mineral density of dentine is significantly lower than that of enamel, caries spreads more extensively

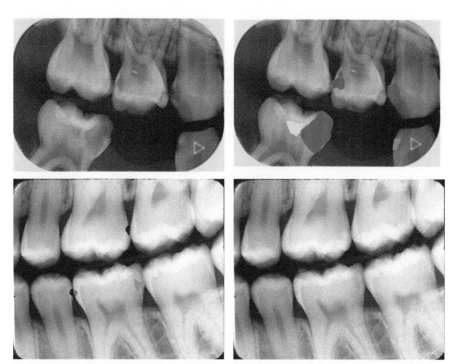

Fig. 1. Bitewings for primary and permanent dentition showing occlusal and proximal caries with various depths. Lesions as are labeled as follows: yellow (occlusal caries), red (proximal caries that extends less than halfway through the thickness of enamel), blue (proximal caries that extends greater than halfway through the thickness of enamel, but does NOT involve the DEJ), green (proximal caries that extends to the DEJ or through the DEJ and into the dentin, but does NOT extend through the dentin greater than half the distance toward the pulp), and purple (proximal caries that extends into the dentin greater than half the distance toward the pulp).

when reaching the dentine, resulting in another radiolucent triangle with a broader base at the DEJ.

Posterior bitewings have high specificity when detecting proximal caries confined to the enamel (0.89; 95% CI 0.84, 0.93)[3]; meanwhile, its sensitivity is only marginal (0.47; 95% CI 0.39, 0.55) as carious lesions may not be visualized on bitewings radiographically until at least 40% demineralization has occurred. The sensitivity and specificity of CBCT in detecting proximal caries are 0.68 (95% CI 0.55, 0.89) and 0.88 (95% CI 0.80, 0.93) respectively.[3]

Occlusal caries
Occlusal enamel caries is mainly diagnosed through clinical examination and may become radiographically evident only when the lesion reaches the DEJ. After thorough cleaning and drying of the teeth, even early incipient caries on the occlusal surfaces can be clearly diagnosed with visual and tactile examination. Bitewing radiographs are not appropriate for diagnosing such early lesions, as they can be easily masked by the buccolingual thickness of the tooth enamel. However, posterior bitewings are still useful for evaluating the extent of occlusal dentinal caries, bearing in mind that carious lesions are usually clinically more advanced than what they appear on radiograph.

CBCT was reported to be slightly more accurate in diagnosing occlusal caries compared with intraoral radiographs given the three-dimensional images generated (sensitivity, 0.76; 95% CI 0.55, 0.89; specificity, 0.54; 95% CI 0.31, 0.75).[3] However, the results have to be interpreted with cautions as most studies were performed in vitro. The pooled sensitivity and specificity of intraoral radiographs from 43 in vitro and in vivo studies were 0.45 (95% CI 0.35, 0.54) and 0.88 (95% CI 0.80, 0.93) respectively.[3]

Facial and lingual/palatal caries
Intraoral radiographs have limited usage in diagnosing smooth surface caries, given the thickness of the tooth itself. Lesions will only be identifiable as they further advance to reach the dentine, producing a well-defined ovoid radiolucent area on the crown.

Recurrent caries
Bitewings play an excellent role in identifying caries underneath a restoration, whereas the performance of CBCT is significantly undermined when detecting recurrent caries beneath restorations. CBCT images are prone to scatter artifacts from attenuation effects related to dental restorations, which may result in marked image degradation and interfere with caries detection.

Root caries
Root caries is on the increase as the population grows older and tends to retain more natural teeth. Periodontal disease could result in root exposure and increased incidence of root caries. Root surface caries is detected clinically; if it occurred on proximal surfaces then imaging may help in the detection of the lesion as an adjunct to clinical examination. Other methods including laser fluorescence have proved to outperform radiographic evaluation of proximal root caries in vitro.[4]

Rampant caries/Radiation caries
Rapidly progressing carious destruction of teeth is called rampant caries. Rampant caries is usually seen in children with poor dietary and oral hygiene habits or adults with xerostomia. Therapeutic radiation to the head and neck is one of the etiologies that induces xerostomia, which can result in a rampant destruction of the teeth. Carious lesions in radiation caries begin at the cervical region and aggressively involve all other surfaces of the crown. The radiographic appearance of radiation caries includes radiolucent areas appearing at the necks of teeth, most obvious on the mesial and distal aspects.

Radiographic mimics of caries
Mach band effect is an optical illusion that contributes to false-positive outcome in caries detection on radiographs. It presents as a more radiolucent region immediately adjacent to the enamel due to the sharply defined density difference between enamel and dentin. The perceived radiolucency caused this phenomenon might be misinterpreted as caries, but the effect will disappear when the light area is masked.

Cervical burnout refers to the diffuse relatively radiolucent area on proximal surfaces at the cervical regions between the cementoenamel junction and the crest of the alveolar ridge. This appearance is the result of the thinner less dense nature if that area which results in decreased x-ray absorption. This phenomenon should not be confused with root surface caries. The cervical root outline will be intact and discernible in cervical burn out, but it will be missing or rough when destroyed by caries. Cervical burnout will usually show a slightly more diffuse, rounded inner border than a carious lesion where tooth substance has been lost.

Non-carious lesions

Definition
Non-carious tooth loss refers to the irreversible structural loss that is not caused by caries. Etiology could be direct tooth-to-tooth contact in attrition, an external object in abrasion, tensile stress from non-axial cyclic loading in abfraction or non-bacteriogenic acid in erosion.[5,6]

Imaging techniques and findings
The radiographic appearances of these entities correspond to the distribution and morphologic changes of the crowns related to the specific etiology (**Fig. 2**A, B). Teeth affected by attrition have flat occlusal planes as opposed to the normal curved surface, and so they tend to become shorter. The pulp chamber and canal could potentially become narrower due to the deposition of secondary dentin. Changes related to abrasion may appear as localized, well-defined, radiolucent lesions at the cervical areas of the affected teeth.

Resorptive Lesions

Definition
Resorption is defined as a process of loss of tooth structure, which can occur within cementum and dentine.[7] This process can be either physiologic or pathologic. Physiologic resorption occurs in deciduous dentition, whereas pathologic resorption occurs mainly in permanent dentition.

External and internal root resorption refer to two distinct processes that involve the breakdown and loss of dental root structure. External root resorption occurs when the external surface of the tooth root is affected often due to factors such as trauma, orthodontic tooth movement, or chronic inflammation. External cervical resorption (ECR) is regarded as one of the most destructive resorptive lesions that impact the cervical region of a tooth and typically exhibits an aggressive nature. Although the exact cause of ECR remains unclear, several predisposing factors have been strongly linked to its occurrence, such as dental trauma, orthodontic procedures, and internal bleaching of endodontically treated teeth.[8]

On the other hand, internal root resorption is a less common condition that takes place within the dental pulp chamber or root canal system. It is characterized by the resorption of dentin from the inside of the tooth, usually as a result of chronic inflammation, infection, or trauma.

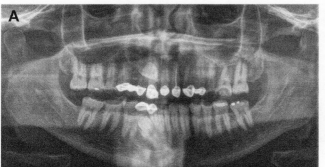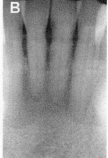

Fig. 2. (*A*) Panoramic radiographs showing signs of generalized dental erosion. (*B*) Periapical radiographs demonstrating attrition of the mandibular incisors. (*Courtesy of* Dr Galal Omami, BDS, MSc, MDentSc, FRCD(C); Lexington, KY, USA).

Imaging techniques and findings

Radiographic signs of external root resorption include irregular root contours, shortened roots, and sometimes, a radiolucent area on the affected root (**Fig. 3**A). For ECR lesions, relying solely on intraoral radiographs may result in inaccurate diagnoses and potentially inappropriate treatment plans as intraoral radiographs might not be able to determine the size and extent of the lesion. Internal root resorption presents as a round or oval radiolucent area within the root canal, often with a distinct outline (see **Fig. 3**B).

The American Association of Endodontists (AAE) and American Academy of Oral and Maxillofacial Radiology (AAOMR) Joint Position Statement on the Use of Cone Beam Computed Tomography in Endodontics lists resorptive lesions as a special condition in which "limited FOV CBCT is the imaging modality of choice in the localization and differentiation of external and internal resorptive defects and the determination of appropriate treatment and prognosis" (**Fig. 4**A, B).[9]

Congenital anomalies of teeth number

Hypodontia

Hypodontia is a common developmental anomaly characterized by the congenital absence of one or more permanent teeth. It is typically diagnosed when a permanent tooth fails to develop and emerge within the expected timeframe.[10] Hypodontia often exhibits a familial tendency, indicating a genetic etiology. Mutations in genes involved in tooth development, such as PAX9 and MSX1, have been associated with hypodontia, and various single nucleotide polymorphisms have been linked with the risk and severity of hypodontia.[11] Environmental factors during prenatal or early postnatal

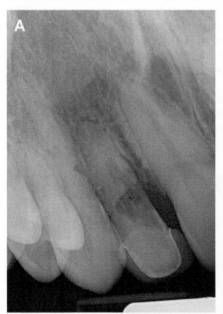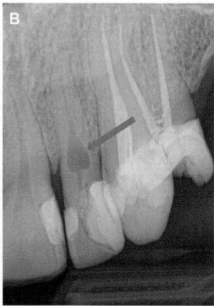

Fig. 3. (*A*) Periapical radiograph showing signs of external root resorption of the maxillary right lateral incisor (*arrow*), whereas (*B*) demonstrates internal resorption of the maxillary left lateral incisor (*arrow*). Note the oval radiolucent area within the root canal with a distinct outline indicating internal root resorption. (*Courtesy of* Dr Galal Omami, BDS, MSc, MDentSc, FRCD(C); Lexington, KY, USA).

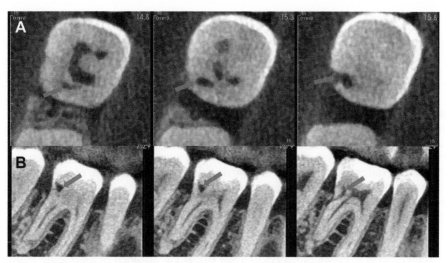

Fig. 4. Axial (*A*) and bucco-lingual views (*B*) from a CBCT volume demonstrating external cervical root resorption of the mandibular right first molar (*arrows*).

stages, such as infections, nutritional deficiencies, trauma, exposure to certain medications, toxins, or radiation during pregnancy can interfere with normal tooth development and increase the risk of hypodontia.[12]

The term "syndromic hypodontia" is used to describe the occurrence of hypodontia as a component of a unique syndrome or in association with a specific signaling pathway related to one or more syndromes. Examples of syndromic hypodontia include ectodermal dysplasia (mutations in EDA, EDAR, and EDARADD genes), Down syndrome (trisomy 21), and various syndromes related to the Wnt signaling pathway, epidermal growth factor (EGF) signaling pathway, and fibroblast growth factor receptor signaling pathway.[13]

Various classification systems have been proposed to categorize hypodontia based on the number and location of missing teeth including the aplasia, oligodontia, anodontia index and the hypodontia anomalies index. The severity of hypodontia is often classified as mild, moderate, or severe, depending on the number and significance of missing teeth.

Hyperdontia

Hyperdontia, also known as supernumerary teeth, is a dental anomaly characterized by the presence of extra teeth beyond the normal dentition. It is a relatively rare condition that can present challenges in terms of oral health, esthetics, and function. Hyperdontia can exhibit a familial predisposition, indicating a genetic component in its etiology. Mutations in certain genes, such as MSX1 and PAX9, have been associated with supernumerary tooth formation.[14] Hyperdontia might be a component of some genetic syndromes, including cleidocranial dysplasia and Gardner syndrome. Environmental factors during prenatal or early postnatal stages, such as trauma, infections, or disruptions in dental follicle development, can contribute to the formation of supernumerary teeth.[15]

Supernumerary teeth can be classified based on their shape and location into.

- *Supplemental teeth* resemble normal teeth and appear alongside the regular dentition.

- *Conical supernumerary teeth* have a simple, cone-shaped structure and are commonly found in the anterior region of the maxilla.
- *Tuberculate supernumerary teeth* are more complex in structure, with multiple cusps or tubercles, and may be found in various locations within the dental arch.
- *Distomolars/paramolars* typically develop in the posterior region of the mouth, and they are more commonly seen in the maxilla.[16]

Imaging techniques and findings for congenital anomalies of teeth number

Intraoral radiographs can provide detailed information about the presence or absence of permanent teeth and their developmental stage, as well as the presence, number, and morphology of supernumerary teeth and their impact on surrounding structures. Panoramic radiography provides an overview of the entire dentition, allowing for the detection of missing or extra teeth, tooth size discrepancies, and abnormalities in tooth development. CBCT provides three-dimensional images of the jaws and teeth, allowing for precise visualization of missing and supernumerary teeth, their positions, and associated structures (**Fig. 5**A, B). It is particularly useful in complex cases, and when dental implants planning or orthodontic treatment is required.

Radiographs in cases of hypodontia will reveal the absence of permanent teeth. Adjacent teeth may exhibit positional changes, such as tipping, rotation, or drifting, due to the space created by the missing tooth. The absence of teeth can lead to alveolar bone atrophy in the affected areas. Findings from radiographic imaging related to supernumerary teeth involve the number and location of these teeth, their shape and composition, their placement and alignment, as well as their impact on neighboring teeth (eg, root resorption). If supernumerary teeth are unerupted, radiographs may provide insights into the position and trajectory of impacted teeth as well as ruling out any associated pathologies.

Congenital anomalies of teeth size

Microdontia

Microdontia is a dental anomaly characterized by the presence of abnormally small teeth. Most commonly affected teeth are the maxillary lateral incisors, maxillary third molars, and supernumerary teeth. Certain syndromes, including ectodermal dysplasia and Down syndrome, are associated with a higher incidence of microdontia. Environmental factors, such as prenatal or postnatal infections, trauma, nutritional deficiencies, or exposure to radiation, can interfere with tooth development and result in microdontia. Microdontia can also be associated with systemic conditions such as hypopituitarism and congenital hypothyroidism.[17]

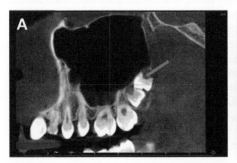 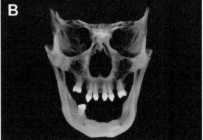

Fig. 5. (*A*) A sagittal cut showing a distomolar (*arrow*), and (*B*) a volume rendered model exhibiting oligodontia in an ectodermal dysplasia patient

True microdontia is characterized by teeth that are significantly smaller than normal, either uniformly throughout the dentition or localized to specific teeth. Relative microdontia is a term used when the size of teeth appears small due to adjacent teeth being larger than average or because of tooth malformation or an oversized dental arch.

Macrodontia

Macrodontia is a dental anomaly characterized by the presence of abnormally large teeth. It is a relatively uncommon condition that can affect the primary or permanent dentition. When localized, it usually is seen with mandibular third molars. Certain syndromes, including Sotos syndrome and hemifacial hypertrophy, are associated with a higher incidence of macrodontia.[18] Environmental factors, such as prenatal or postnatal infections, or maternal hormonal disturbances might prolong or increase the activity of dental lamina leading to macrodontia. Macrodontia can also be associated with systemic conditions such as gigantism.[19]

IMAGING TECHNIQUES AND FINDINGS IN CONGENITAL ANOMALIES OF TEETH SIZE

Periapical radiographs assist in identifying the extent of microdontia/ macrodontia and its impact on adjacent teeth and supporting structures (**Fig. 6**A). Bitewing radiographs assist in evaluating the size discrepancies between affected teeth and adjacent teeth, as well as assessing any spacing issues or alignment problems caused by microdontia. Panoramic radiographs aid in assessing the overall size, shape, and alignment of teeth affected by microdontia/macrodontia, as well as their relationship to adjacent structures (see **Fig. 6**B).

Congenital Anomalies of Teeth Form and Structure

Localized processes

Gemination and fusion. Gemination is a rare dental anomaly that occurs during tooth development, in which a single tooth bud attempts to divide into two separate teeth.[20] This process results in the formation of a tooth with a large, bifid crown or, in rare cases, complete division throughout the crown and root. On the other hand, fusion

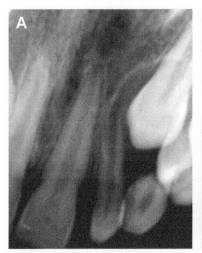
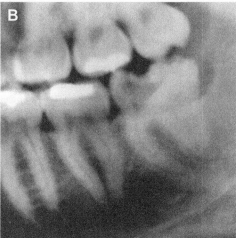

Fig. 6. (*A*) A periapical image of a microdontic maxillary left lateral incisor and (*B*) is a cropped panoramic image that shows a macrodontic mandibular left third molar.

of teeth results from the combining of adjacent tooth germs, resulting in union of the developing teeth. It also presents as a larger than normal size crown, often with two separate roots.[21,22] The number of teeth present in the dental arch is important to help differentiate fusion from gemination. In fusion, there is a reduction in the tooth count, whereas in gemination, the tooth count remains normal (**Fig. 7**). Both phenomena are more common in primary teeth; fusion is also more common in the anterior teeth. Limited field-of-view (FOV) CBCT should be considered for preoperative assessment of geminated/fused teeth if endodontic therapy was needed because of their complex morphology.[9]

Concrescence. Concrescence involves the fusion of two or more teeth by their cementum, most often the maxillary molars.[23] It is very difficult, if not impossible, to distinguish concrescence from superimposition on two-dimensional radiographs. Supplemental projections with different angles or CBCT might be needed for better delineation of anatomy of roots involved (**Fig. 8**).[24]

Taurodontism. Taurodontism is characterized by an enlargement of the pulp chamber and apical displacement of the floor of the pulp chamber in multi-rooted teeth, most commonly the molars. In taurodontism, the crown appears normal, but the roots are shortened, and the pulp chamber is enlarged, extending into the root area (**Fig. 9**). This results in a tooth with a large pulp chamber, small root canals, and shorter roots, which can cause complications during dental procedures such as root canal treatments and extractions.[25–27]

Dens invaginatus. Dens invaginatus, also known as dens in dente, is characterized by an infolding of the outer surface into the interior of a tooth. The maxillary lateral incisors followed by maxillary central incisors are commonly affected. If it happens coronally, it caused by infolding of the enamel organ producing an invagination within the body of the tooth, which becomes lined with enamel.[28] This invagination can vary in depth, ranging from a mild groove on the tooth surface to an extensive channel extending into the pulp chamber. The radicular type is the result of an invagination of Hertwig's epithelial root sheath and is lined by cementum.[29] Most cases are discovered radiographically by identifying the radiopaque enamel lining. Radicular invagination may appear as poorly defined lucent areas running longitudinally within the root. Depending on the severity of presentation, limited FOV CBCT should be considered for preoperative assessment of affected teeth if endodontic therapy or apical surgery was to be performed[9,30,31] (**Fig. 10A–C**).

Dens evaginatus. In contrast to dens invaginatus, dens evaginatus is the result of an outfolding of the enamel organ, creating an enamel tubercle or accessory cusp. The

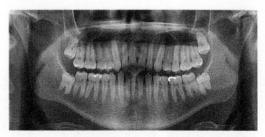

Fig. 7. A panoramic radiograph that shows fusion between the mandibular left central and lateral incisors. (*Courtesy of* Dr Galal Omami, BDS, MSc, MDentSc, FRCD(C); Lexington, KY, USA).

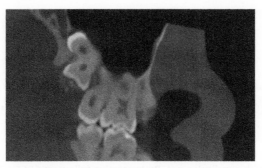

Fig. 8. A sagittal view of a CBCT scan demonstrating concrescence between the roots of the maxillary third molar and distomolar. (*Courtesy of* Dr Galal Omami, BDS, MSc, MDentSc, FRCD(C); Lexington, KY, USA).

mandibular premolars are affected most frequently. Imaging may help demonstrate how much dentin and possibly if a pulp horn is extending into the tubercle.[32]

Dilaceration. Dilaceration is a dental anomaly characterized by an abnormal angulation or curvature in the root or crown of a tooth. This distortion can occur during tooth development and may affect the tooth's shape, position, and eruption pattern. Radiographs provide the best means of detecting a radicular dilaceration (**Fig. 11**). On a two-dimensional radiograph, if the direction of the curve was either buccal or lingual, the apical part of the root may appear as a round radiopaque area with a central radiolucency (the apical foramen) and surrounded by the radiolucent periodontal lingament (PDL) space, giving a bull's eye appearance.[33]

Enamel pearl. An enamel pearl is a small, spherical nodule of ectopic enamel that develops on the root's surface, typically near the cementoenamel junction or at the furcation area. Enamel pearls may have a core of dentin and, rarely, even pulp tissue. On radiographs, enamel pearls appear smooth, round, and have enamel radiopacity (**Fig. 12**).[34,35]

Turner's hypoplasia
Turner's hypoplasia is a local defect in the crown of a permanent tooth as a result of infection or trauma to the deciduous predecessor. The crown morphologic irregularities are often evident on radiographs. Hypoplastic area may appear radiolucent depending the degree of hypomineralization.[36]

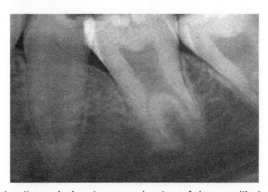

Fig. 9. A periapical radiograph showing taurodontism of the mandibular first molar.

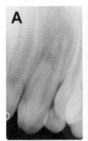
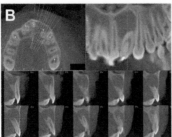
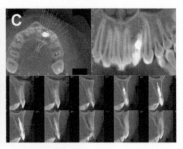

Fig. 10. A preoperative periapical radiograph (*A*) and CBCT (*B*) that show a dense in dente that is associated with a radicular cyst. Postoperative follow-up CBCT (*C*) shows healing of the apical area.

REGIONAL AND GENERALIZED DISEASES
Hereditary Amelogenesis Imperfecta

Amelogenesis imperfecta (AI) refers to a heterogenous hereditary group of conditions associated with qualitative and quantitative defects of the enamel. The estimated prevalence varies from 1 in 700 to 1:14,000 globally.[37]

Many classifications and subclassifications exist for grouping AI with different phenotypes and genetic causes. But in general, AI can be classified into four main types, including (1) hypoplastic, (2) hypomaturation AI, (3) hypocalcified AI, and (4) hypomaturation- hypoplastic with taurodontism.[38]

Hypoplastic AI is a quantitative defect occurs due to disturbances occurred when ameloblasts deposit organic matrix during enamel formation.[38,39] The affected teeth may appear smaller, with thinner or pitted enamel. Radiographically, the enamel layer appears thinner, but the radiodensity appears similar to that of the normal enamel. As the quality of enamel is not affected in hypoplasia, adhesive restorations can be used for restorative treatments (**Fig. 13**).

Hypocalcified AI occurs when the mineralization of the enamel matrix deposited by the ameloblasts is being affected.[38] The enamel is of normal thickness, but the quality is severely affected, appearing yellowish and soft.[38,39] The enamel may suffer from posteruptive breakdown or easily scrapped away by sharp instruments. Patients may be hypersensitive to tooth brushing or cold food.[37] Radiographically, hypocalcified AI

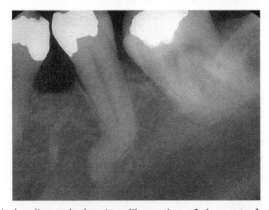

Fig. 11. A periapical radiograph showing dilaceration of the root of mandibular second premolar.

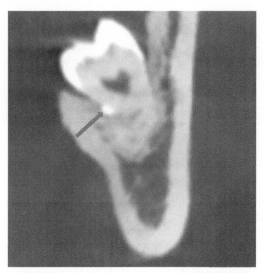

Fig. 12. A cross-sectional CBCT view showing an enamel pearl (*arrow*) on the lingual surface of the mandibular molar. (*Courtesy of* Dr Galal Omami, BDS, MSc, MDentSc, FRCD(C); Lexington, KY, USA).

displayed the lowest mean and maximum enamel density, and its radiodensity is even more radiolucent than dentine (**Fig. 14**A, B).[39,40]

Hypomatured Al manifests due to defects occurred in the enlargement and maturation of enamel crystals in the enamel matrix dentine.[39,40] The enamel appears mottled, relatively soft and easily chipped away. The enamel radiodensity of hypomatured Al is more radiolucent than normal enamel, but more radiopaque than hypocalcified Al and

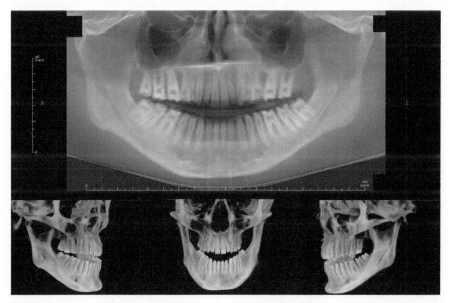

Fig. 13. A reconstructed panoramic view and volume rendered models that demonstrate the smaller crowns and generalized diastema in a hypoplastic amelogenesis imperfecta patient.

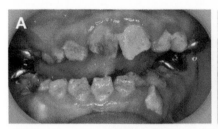
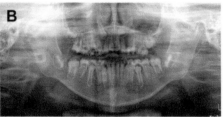

Fig. 14. An intraoral photograph (*A*) and a panoramic radiograph (*B*) for a patient with the hypocalcified variant of amelogenesis imperfecta demonstrating the soft yellow enamel that appears to be as or less dense than dentin radiographically.

similar to dentine. The enamel thickness is unaffected, even though posteruptive breakdown may occur.[39,40]

Hypomaturative-hypoplastic AI with taurodontism is subtype of AI with enamel displaying both defects in thickness and texture. The enamel appears soft, mottled with a yellow-brown or opaque hue and with pits or thinner. The condition is often associated with taurodontism in the molars.[37]

The diagnosis of AI is mainly clinical, and radiographs are used for special investigations to verify the diagnosis and other associated conditions. A detailed family history is also important to identify the hereditary patterns.

Hereditary Dentine Disorder

Dentinogenesis imperfecta

Dentinogenesis imperfecta type 1 (DGI-I) is associated with osteogenesis imperfecta (OI). Other than the bone and dentine, other body structure rich in collagen, including skin and sclera might be affected. Diagnosis of DGI-I is mainly based on the medical history of OI and clinical findings. The teeth appear either amber-brown in color or with blue-grayish hue due to deposition of other minerals at the defective dentine (**Fig. 15**A, B).[37] The quality and thickness of enamel is normal, but due to defects at the DEJ, it is highly susceptible to wear, fracture, and caries after dentine exposure.[38] Radiographically, pulpal obliteration is often detected; in severe cases, complete pulp obliteration might even be noticeable before eruption. Other than OI, DGI can also manifest in other syndromes associated with connective tissue and joint disorders, for instance,

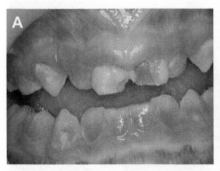
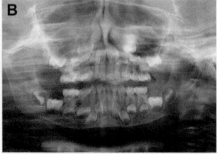

Fig. 15. An intraoral photograph (*A*) and a panoramic radiograph (*B*) for a type I dentinogenesis imperfecta patient demonstrating the amber-brown colored teeth, the bulbous crowns, and the obliteration of the pulp radiographically.

Ehlers-Danlos syndrome, Goldblatt syndrome, Schimke immuno-osseous dysplasia, and Bruck syndrome.[41]

In both DGI type I and II, the affected teeth appear amber or greyish. The crowns look bulbous due to cervical constrictions and short roots.[41–43] Enamel thickness and density are unaffected but chip off very easily due to defective enamel–dentine junction. The dental pulp may be obliterated due to continuous dentine breakdown.[37]

DGI type III (MIM 125500) is mainly reported in Maryland, USA; in a town called Brandywine habituated with a multiracial population mainly constituted of Native Americans, African American, and Caucasians.[37] The condition affects both primary and permanent dentition, with opalescent appearance ranging from amber to greyish blue color resemble the appearance of DGI-I and II.[41–43] Owing to severe hypotrophy of the dentine, the affected teeth appear hollow with enlarged pulp.[37] Frequent pulpal exposure often found in the affected primary teeth.

Dentin dysplasia

Dentin dysplasia can be subclassified into type I radicular dentin dysplasia which the dental roots are predominantly affected and type II coronal dentin dysplasia, where the defects are mainly present at the coronal part of the affected teeth.

The reported prevalence of type I radicular dentin dysplasia (DD) (MIM 125400) is 1:10,000.[42] In type I radicular DD, the dental roots of affected teeth in general will appear shorter and more bulbous than normal, although in some subdivision the root can be completely absent with concurrent radiolucency (**Fig. 16**).[44] Complete or partial pulp with a semilunar pulp chamber is often found in both primary and permanent teeth in DD-I.[42] Although the coronal structure is minimally affected in radicular DD, the crowns are more prone to fracture, excessive mobility and premature exfoliation due to defective dental roots.[42] Periapical radiolucency is a common finding under the apparently sound crown.[42]

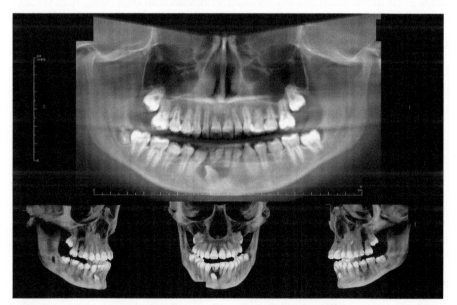

Fig. 16. A reconstructed panoramic view and volume rendered models that demonstrate the shorter underdeveloped roots in a type I radicular dentin dysplasia. Incidentally, the impacted mandibular right canine is associated with a dentigerous cyst.

For type II coronal DD (MIM 125420), the primary dentition is more severely affected than the permanent dentition.[43] The deciduous crowns of coronal DD appear short and bulbous, discolored with a brownish translucent hue, and very prone to wearing.[43] Radiographically, the coronal pulp is usually obliterated. For the permanent teeth, the color appears less abnormal with occasional brownish or greyish discoloration. Pulp obliteration is also observed but to a lesser extent, giving a classical presentation of "thistle-shape" pulp chamber, which a comparatively large pulp chamber is found with long narrow root canals.[43]

Regional odontodysplasia

Regional odontodysplasia or "ghost teeth" refers to a rare localized condition where both the enamel and dentine of a few teeth in the dentition are severely malformed. As both the enamel and dentine are markedly hypoplastic and poorly mineralized, radiographic projections of these teeth will result in ambiguous images with ill-defined distinction between the enamel and dentine, thus being called as "ghost teeth".[45] The pulp chamber is usually enlarged with open apices and coronal pulpal calcification observed.[46] Conventional radiography aids in the initial investigation of unerupted teeth and appreciation of the radiodensity of the affected tooth structures,[47,48] allowing clinicians to make differential diagnosis. From previous case report, CBCT can demonstrate the radiodensity of the affected teeth in comparisons with the unaffected neighboring dentition.[47,48]

SUMMARY

A thorough clinical evaluation is needed before determining imaging needs for patients with acquired or congenital abnormalities of teeth. Properly acquired bitewings are the imaging standard of care for posterior interproximal caries detection. Both two-dimensional and three-dimensional imaging play a significant role not only in the detection but also in treatment planning and management of congenital dental anomalies. Some of the dental anomalies are identified as incidental findings during routine radiographic examination, so a thorough and systematic radiographic evaluation is necessary.

CLINICS CARE POINTS

- A thorough clinical evaluation is needed before determining imaging needs for patients with acquired or congenital abnormalities of teeth.
- Properly acquired bitewings as the imaging standard of care for posterior caries detection.
- Both two-dimensional and three-dimensional imaging play a significant role not only in the detection but also in treatment planning and management of congenital dental anomalies.
- Some of the dental anomalies are identified as incidental findings during routine radiographic examination, so a thorough and systematic radiographic evaluation is necessary.

DISCLOSURE

None of the authors have any commercial or financial conflicts of interest and any funding sources.

REFERENCES

1. Machiulskiene V, Campus G, Carvalho JC, et al. Terminology of dental caries and dental caries management: consensus report of a workshop organized by ORCA and Cariology Research Group of IADR. Caries Res 2020;54(1):7–14.

2. Radiation Protection 172. Cone beam Ct for dental and maxillofacial radiology: evidence based guidelines. 2012. Available at: https://ec.europa.eu/energy/sites/ener/files/documents/172.pdf.

3. Walsh T, Macey R, Riley P, et al. Imaging modalities to inform the detection and diagnosis of early caries. Cochrane Database Syst Rev 2021;(3). https://doi.org/10.1002/14651858.CD014545.

4. Göstemeyer G, Preus M, Elhennawy K, et al. Accuracy of different approaches for detecting proximal root caries lesions in vitro. Clin Oral Invest 2023;27(3):1143–51.

5. Warreth A, Abuhijleh E, Almaghribi MA, et al. Tooth surface loss: A review of literature. The Saudi dental journal 2020;32(2):53–60.

6. Carvalho TS, Colon P, Ganss C, et al. Consensus report of the European Federation of Conservative Dentistry: erosive tooth wear—diagnosis and management. Clin Oral Invest 2015;19:1557–61.

7. Machiulskiene V, Campus G, Carvalho JC, et al. Terminology of dental caries and dental caries management: consensus report of a workshop organized by ORCA and Cariology Research Group of IADR. Caries Res 2020;54(1):7–14.

8. Heithersay G. Management of tooth resorption. Aust Dent J 2007;52:S105–21.

9. Fayad MI, Nair M, Levin MD, et al. AAE and AAOMR joint position statement: use of cone beam computed tomography in endodontics 2015 update. Oral surgery, oral medicine, oral pathology and oral radiology 2015;120(4):508–12.

10. Kielan-Grabowska Z, Kawala B, Antoszewska-Smith J. Hypodontia–not only an orthodontic problem. Dent Med Probl 2019;56(4):373–7.

11. Yu M, Wong SW, Han D, et al. Genetic analysis: Wnt and other pathways in non-syndromic tooth agenesis. Oral Dis 2019;25(3):646–51.

12. Al-Ani AH, Antoun JS, Thomson WM, et al. Hypodontia: an update on its etiology, classification, and clinical management. BioMed Res Int 2017;2017.

13. Doolan B, Onoufriadis A, Kantaputra P, et al. WNT10A, dermatology and dentistry. Br J Dermatol 2021;185(6):1105–11.

14. Wang Y, Kong H, Mues G, et al. Msx1 mutations: how do they cause tooth agenesis? J Dent Res 2011;90(3):311–6.

15. Cammarata-Scalisi F, Avendaño A, Callea M. Main genetic entities associated with supernumerary teeth. Arch Argent Pediatr 2018;116(6):437–44.

16. Suljkanovic N, Balic D, Begic N. Supernumerary and supplementary teeth in a non-syndromic patients. Med Arch 2021;75(1):78.

17. Neville BW, Damm DD, Allen CM, et al. Color atlas of oral and maxillofacial diseases-E-book. Elsevier Health Sciences; 2018.

18. Chetty M, Beshtawi K, Roomaney I, et al. MACRODONTIA: A brief overview and a case report of KBG syndrome. Radiology Case Reports 2021;16(6):1305–10.

19. Mainali A, Denny C, Sumanth K, et al. Non syndromic generalised macrodontia. Journal of Nepal Dental Association 2010;11(2):150–3.

20. Shah P, Chander JM, Noar J, et al. Management of 'double teeth'in children and adolescents. Int J Paediatr Dent 2012;22(6):419–26.

21. Vegh T. Gemination and fusion. Oral Surg Oral Med Oral Pathol 1975;40(6):816–7.

22. Parks C. Fusion and gemination. Oral Surg Oral Med Oral Pathol 1970;29(3):394.

23. Sugiyama M, Ogawa I, Suei Y, et al. Concrescence of teeth: cemental union between the crown of an impacted tooth and the roots of an erupted tooth. J Oral Pathol Med 2007;36(1):60–2.

24. Syed AZ, Alluri LC, Mallela D, et al. Concrescence: cone-beam computed tomography imaging perspective. Case reports in dentistry, 2016, 2016.

25. Jafarzadeh H, Azarpazhooh A, Mayhall J. Taurodontism: a review of the condition and endodontic treatment challenges. Int Endod J 2008;41(5):375–88.

26. Metgud S, Metgud R, Rani K. Management of a patient with a taurodont, single-rooted molars associated with multiple dental anomalies: a spiral computerized tomography evaluation. Oral Surg Oral Med Oral Pathol Oral Radiol Endod 2009;108(2):e81–6.

27. MacDonald D. Taurodontism. Review. Oral Radiol 2020;36(2):129–32.

28. Zhang C, Hou BX. [Reconsideration of the diagnosis and treatment for dens invaginatus]. Zhonghua Kou Qiang Yi Xue Za Zhi 2020;55(5):302–8.

29. Verma S, Dasukil S, Namdev Sable M, et al. Radicular variant of dens in dente (RDinD) in a patient undergoing radioisotope therapy. Journal of Taibah University Medical Sciences 2022;17(6):1094–8.

30. McClammy TV. Endodontic applications of cone beam computed tomography. Dent Clin North Am 2014;58(3):545–59.

31. Dos Santos GNA, Sousa-Neto MD, de Assis HC, et al. Prevalence and morphological analysis of dens invaginatus in anterior teeth using cone beam computed tomography: A systematic review and meta-analysis. Arch Oral Biol 2023;105715.

32. Dankner E, Harari D, Rotstein I. Dens evaginatus of anterior teeth: Literature review and radiographic survey of 15,000 teeth. Oral Surgery, Oral Medicine, Oral Pathology, Oral Radiology, and Endodontology 1996;81(4):472–5.

33. Jafarzadeh H, Abbott PV. Dilaceration: review of an endodontic challenge. J Endod 2007;33(9):1025–30.

34. Moskow BS, Canut PM. Studies on root enamel: (2) Enamel pearls. A review of their morphology, localization, nomenclature, occurrence, classification, histogenesis and incidence. J Clin Periodontol 1990;17(5):275–81.

35. Zengin AZ, Sumer AP, Ozturk G, et al. Imaging characteristics of enamel pearls on CBCT and their co-relation with supernumerary tooth. Oral Radiol 2021;1–8.

36. Via WF Jr. Enamel defects induced by trauma during tooth formation. Oral Surg Oral Med Oral Pathol 1968;25(1):49–54.

37. Schuurs AHB, Matos T. Pathology of the hard dental tissues. Wiley-Blackwell; 2013.

38. Witkop CJ Jr. Amelogenesis imperfecta, dentinogenesis imperfecta and dentin dysplasia revisited: problems in classification. J Oral Pathol 1988;17(9–10): 547–53.

39. Aldred MJ, Savarirayan R, Crawford PJ. Amelogenesis imperfecta: a classification and catalogue for the 21st century. Oral Dis 2003;9(1):19–23.

40. Wright JT, Torain M, Long K, et al. Amelogenesis imperfecta: genotype-phenotype studies in 71 families. Cells Tissues Organs 2011;194(2–4):279–83.

41. Barron MJ, McDonnell ST, Mackie I, et al. Hereditary dentine disorders: dentinogenesis imperfecta and dentine dysplasia. Orphanet J Rare Dis 2008;3:31.

42. Kim JW, Simmer JP. Hereditary dentin defects. J Dent Res 2007;86(5):392–9.

43. Shields ED, Bixler D, el-Kafrawy AM. A proposed classification for heritable human dentine defects with a description of a new entity. Arch Oral Biol 1973; 18(4):543–53.

44. Chen D, Li X, Lu F, et al. Dentin dysplasia type I-A dental disease with genetic heterogeneity. Oral Dis 2019;25(2):439–46.

45. Nijakowski K, Woś P, Surdacka A. Regional odontodysplasia: a systematic review of case reports. Int J Environ Res Publ Health 2022;19(3). https://doi.org/10.3390/ijerph19031683.

46. Zegarelli EV, Kutscher AH, Applebaum E, et al. Odontodysplasia. Oral surgery, oral medicine, and oral pathotllogy 1963;16:187–93.

47. Damasceno JX, Couto JL, Alves KS, et al. Generalized odontodysplasia in a 5-year-old patient with Hallermann-Streiff syndrome: clinical aspects, cone beam computed tomography findings, and conservative clinical approach. Oral surgery, oral medicine, oral pathology and oral radiology 2014;118(2):e58–64.

48. de Sá Cavalcante D, Fonteles CS, Ribeiro TR, et al. Mandibular Regional Odontodysplasia in an 8-year-old Boy showing Teeth Disorders, Gubernaculum Tracts, and Altered Bone Fractal Pattern. International journal of clinical pediatric dentistry 2018;11(2):128–34.

The Role of Radiographic Imaging in the Diagnosis and Management of Periodontal and Peri-Implant Diseases

Abdo Ismail, DDS, MS[a], Firas Al Yafi, DDS, MS[b],*

KEYWORDS

- Radiography • Cone-beam computed tomography • Periodontitis • Peri-implantitis
- Dental implants

KEY POINTS

- Radiographic imaging serves as an indispensable tool for diagnosing and managing periodontal disease, identifying bone loss, defects, and formulating treatment strategies.
- Radiographic examination plays a crucial role in implant planning, as it is essential for evaluating bone dimensions and ensuring proper implant placement to achieve successful outcomes.
- CBCT provides a comprehensive view of the implant site and becomes especially important when traditional radiographs do not offer sufficient information.
- Radiographs also play a significant role in diagnosing peri-implant diseases, helping identify complications, and enabling timely intervention to preserve the of dental implants.

INTRODUCTION

Periodontal diseases are conditions that affect the periodontium, which comprises the supportive structures surrounding a tooth, including gingival tissue, alveolar bone, cementum, and periodontal ligament.[1] Gingivitis is the milder form of periodontal disease, affecting up to 90% of the population and reversible with improved oral hygiene. On the other hand, periodontitis is a chronic, irreversible, and more severe inflammatory disease state.[1] It is the most prevalent chronic oral disease affecting the adult population in the United States, with 64.7 million (42.7%) American adults diagnosed with mild, moderate, or severe periodontitis.[2] Periodontal disease initiation and propagation is caused by dysbiosis of the commensal oral microbiota present in the dental plaque, which disrupts the balance and interactions with the host's immune defenses,

[a] Private Practice, 726 Crystal Oak Lane, Arlington, TX 76005, USA; [b] Private Practice, Diplomate of the American Board of Periodontology, Arab Board of Oral Surgery, 5625 Saint Thomas Dr, Plano, TX 75094-4617, USA
* Corresponding author. 8000 Coit Road, Suite 200, Plano, TX 75025.
E-mail address: firasyafi@hotmail.com

Dent Clin N Am 68 (2024) 247–258
https://doi.org/10.1016/j.cden.2023.09.002
0011-8532/24/© 2023 Elsevier Inc. All rights reserved.

ultimately leading to inflammation and disease.[3] A comprehensive clinical and radiographic examination is crucial for effectively diagnosing and managing patients with destructive periodontal diseases. Attachment level should be assessed clinically through periodontal probing. However, radiographic examination is still necessary to evaluate bone levels and morphology.[4]

RADIOGRAPHIC IMAGING IN PERIODONTAL DISEASE

Conducting an Initial assessment of periodontal tissues establishes a diagnostic baseline, while periodic evaluations monitor disease progression and treatment outcome.[5,6] Radiography plays a vital role in assessing the status of hard tissues and identifying various pathologies.[5] It also allows for assessing the condition, planning, and executing appropriate treatment.[6] Two-dimensional (2D) radiographic techniques including bitewing, periapical, and panoramic radiographs are commonly employed for the diagnosis of periodontal disease.[7] Panoramic radiographs can be utilized to obtain an overall view of the patient's entire dentition, jaws, and related structures (**Fig. 1**A–C, **2**A–C). Despite the improved image quality of intraoral images, which are typically favored for assessing bone level and morphology, the literature suggests that the panoramic image is sufficient only if supplemented by vertical or horizontal bitewings.[4] The vertical bitewing is the most useful intraoral radiograph (IR) for assessing periodontal disease and bone levels due to its thorough visibility and minimal distortion.[4] 2D radiographs are commonly employed due to their ease of acquisition, cost-effectiveness, and ability to produce high-resolution images.[7] Nevertheless, they come with limitations, including overlapping anatomic structures, challenges in standardization, and potential underestimation of bone defects.[8,9] To overcome the limitations of 2D radiographs, three-dimensional (3D) imaging techniques, such as cone-beam computed tomography (CBCT) are employed. CBCT provides 2D and 3D images essential for diagnosing and planning treatment for intra-bony defects, furcation involvements, and buccal/lingual bone destructions.[8,10] While periapical radiographs are limited in providing information about the extent of furcation bone loss, CBCT images offer high-resolution views that enable accurate assessment of defects, roots involved, and lesion dimensions, making it valuable in evaluating furcations and interradicular bone in periodontics.[11] In cases with extensive bone loss that led to furcation involvement, an accurate diagnosis of interradicular bone loss is an important factor before deciding on the appropriate treatment.[12] Previous studies indicated that CBCT images were more effective in detecting periodontal defects compared to other radiograph types. Furthermore, CBCT showed higher diagnostic accuracy than periapical radiographs in identifying interradicular bone loss.[13,14] Another study concluded that CBCT images of maxillary molars offer comprehensive details on furcation involvement, providing a dependable foundation for making treatment decisions.[11] Additionally, 2D radiographs may not be sufficient in detecting intra-bony alveolar defects because the cortical plate can obstruct changes in spongy bone. Therefore, 3D imaging is necessary to accurately outline the alveolar defects.[8] It can be concluded that CBCT images offer extra details, including the dimensions of bony defects in the buccolingual direction, the number of bony walls present at different levels of the defect, and the presence or absence of dehiscences and/or fenestrations[15,16] (**Fig. 3**A and B).

The 2017 American Academy of Periodontology consensus supports a combination of 2D radiographic series and clinical probing as the gold standard for periodontal evaluation. However, CBCT imaging is recognized as beneficial in specific cases, such as detecting advanced furcation lesions, assessing dental implant options, and diagnosing complex conditions.[17] Ongoing research demonstrates the increasing

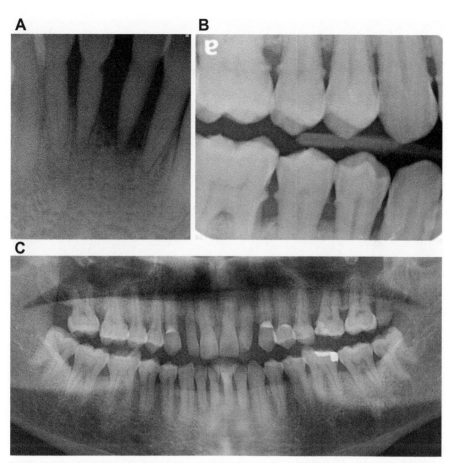

Fig. 1. Conventional 2D Radiographs. (*A*) Periapical view showing severe marginal bone resorption around the mandibular incisors. (*B*) Horizontal bitewing showing generalized interproximal calculus buildup. (*C*) Panoramic view provides a broad view of the dentition and marginal periodontium.

value of CBCT in certain clinical scenarios, providing valuable insights for the profession.[17] More research is needed to validate its benefits and address potential limitations. While offering valuable information, thorough evaluation of the expenses and radiation exposure compared to the conventional radiographs is essential before incorporating CBCT into routine clinical practice.[4,12]

RADIOGRAPHIC IMAGING IN DENTAL IMPLANT

Radiographic examination is a fundamental step in implant planning because it provides essential information about the patient's anatomy, bone quality, and dimensions of the implant site. It helps to determine the most accurate Implant position and plan the procedure accordingly.[18–21] While panoramic and intraoral periapical radiographs can provide valuable information, they have limitations (**Fig. 4**A–C, **5**A and B). 2D imaging can suffer from distortion, magnification, and elongation, which may affect the accuracy of dimensional measurements and can lead to potential errors during treatment planning. CBCT addresses the limitations of 2D imaging and offers superior

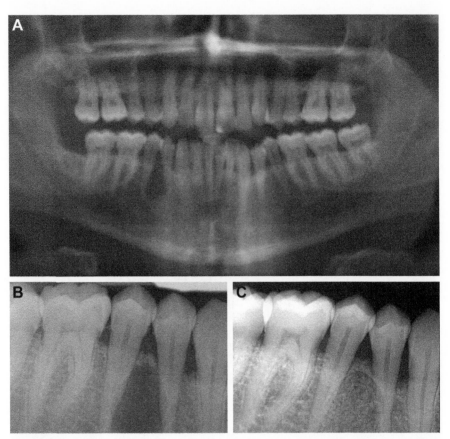

Fig. 2. (*A*) Panoramic view shows a well-defined, radiolucent lesion between the mandibular right premolars. (*B*) Periapical image shows the same lesion. (*C*) Periapical image shows the bone healing 3 months after enucleation and bone grafting. The histologic study revealed a lateral periodontal cyst.

image quality. It provides detailed cross-sectional images that enable precise measurements of alveolar ridge width, height, and angulation.[19,20] CBCT is particularly useful in assessing complex anatomy where accurate measurements are crucial for successful and safe implant placement (**Fig. 6**A–D). Moreover, CBCT when combined with computer guidance is a powerful tool that enhances the entire implant therapy process. It facilitates proper coordination between the diagnostic, surgical, and prosthetic aspects, leading to more predictable outcomes for patients undergoing dental implant treatment[22] (**Fig. 7**A–D, **8**A–E). The choice of radiographic modality for postoperative assessment of dental implants depends on the complexity of the case and the specific clinical circumstances. Intraoral periapical radiographs are suitable for routine assessment of individual implants, while panoramic radiographs can provide an overview of multiple implants. However, in cases of complications like local infection or nerve injury, CBCT imaging is indicated to obtain more detailed information and aid in appropriate management.[23] There is a consensus among dental implant societies that thorough clinical examination and 2D radiographs are the first steps in assessing an implant site.[18–22,24,25] However, when more detailed information is required for complex cases, CBCT is considered superior to 2D radiographs.[19,20,24]

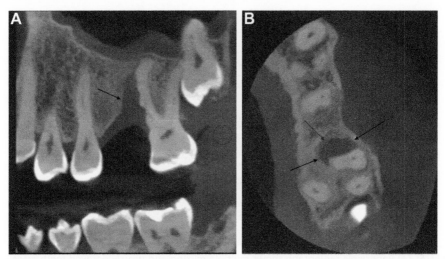

Fig. 3. Limited field-of-view (FOV) CBCT scan. (A) Sagittal CBCT image shows a deep, infrabony defect along the mesial root of the maxillary second M (*arrow*). (B) Axial CBCT section reveals a three-walled vertical defect (*arrow*).

The use of CBCT should be justified based on the individual patient's needs, and radiation dose optimization is essential to minimize risks.[18,20,26] Reviewing the CBCT data by a skilled healthcare provider is also emphasized to ensure accurate interpretation and diagnosis.[18,20,25] Different organizations have specific recommendations for when to use CBCT, with some suggesting it only in critical anatomic situations and guided surgery,[18–20,22,24] while others advocate for its use in most treatment cases.[25]

PERI-IMPLANTITIS

Dental implants are widely regarded as a viable and enduring solution for the replacement of missing teeth.[27] High survival rates, ranging from 95% to 98% over a 10-year period, have been reported.[28] Nevertheless, their utilization is accompanied by a range of complications, with biological complications being the most frequently encountered. These include soft tissue dehiscence, marginal bone loss, peri-implant mucositis, and peri-implantitis.[29] Peri-implantitis refers to a persistent inflammatory condition that leads to the deterioration of the tissues encompassing the dental implant.[30] The

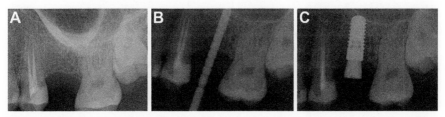

Fig. 4. (A) Periapical view shows the available alveolar bone height and mesiodistal width at the proposed implant site. (B) Radiographic stent indicating the intended implant's mesiodistal angulation and osteotomy depth. (C) Immediate postoperative evaluation of implant placement.

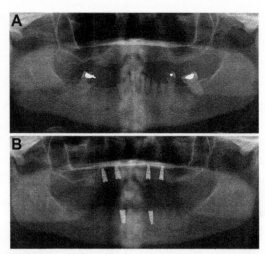

Fig. 5. (*A*) Panoramic radiograph shows multiple missing and grossly decayed teeth associated with generalized alveolar bone resorption. (*B*) Postoperative image showing multiple implant placement in both arches for overdentures.

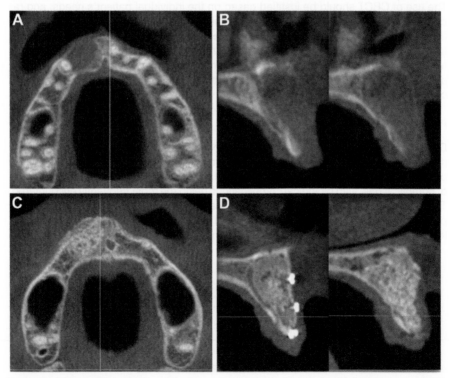

Fig. 6. (*A*) Axial CBCT view shows a large cyst in the right anterior maxilla. (*B*) Cross-sectional CBCT images show the cyst has caused expansion and erosion of the facial plate. (*C* and *D*), Axial and cross-sectional images show bone healing 6 months after a successful guided bone regeneration procedure.

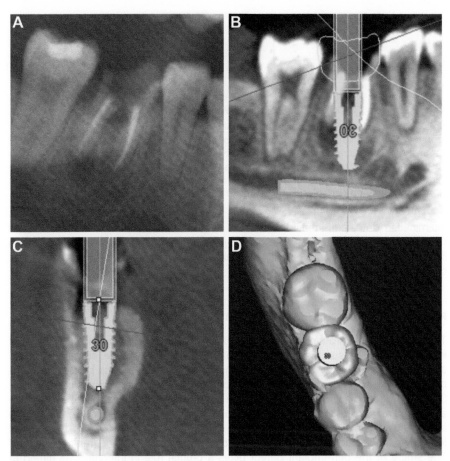

Fig. 7. (*A*) Periapical image shows a non-restorable mandibular first molar. (*B-D*), CBCT images show virtual digital planning taking into consideration the future crown and site anatomy.

prevalence of peri-implantitis varies significantly, spanning from 2.7% to 47.1%. This wide range can be attributed to various etiologic factors and different disease definitions related to peri-implant conditions.[27] Signs of peri-implant tissue inflammation, such as deep probing depth or bleeding upon probing, in conjunction with progressive bone loss, are commonly observed in implants affected by this ailment.[31] Tissue inflammation, which involves symptoms like redness, swelling, and enlargement of the mucosal tissue, is commonly observed in both peri-implant mucositis and peri-implantitis. However, the key distinguishing factor for peri-implantitis is the presence of radiographic bone loss.[32] Previous study by Derks and colleagues (2016) demonstrated that peri-implantitis might develop soon after implant placement. Fifty-two percent of the implants showed early signs of bone loss (>0.5 mm) after the second year of placement, while 66% of implants exhibited bone loss after the third year in function.[33] The 2017 world workshop established that peri-implantitis diagnosis requires the presence of bleeding and/or suppuration on gentle probing, increased probing depth compared to previous examinations, and bone loss beyond crestal bone level changes resulting from initial bone remodeling.[34] In the absence of previous

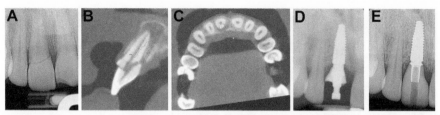

Fig. 8. (*A*) Periapical image shows a horizontal fracture in the maxillary right central incisor caused by a traumatic injury. (*B*) Cross-sectional CBCT image provides additional details about the buccal bone and root position in the alveolar bone. (*C*) Axial CBCT section demonstrates bucco-palatal position of the proposed implant site. (*D*) Immediate postoperative periapical view showing placed implant with a customized healing abutment attached. (*E*) 13-month follow-up periapical view demonstrating crestal bone stability.

examination data, peri-implantitis can be diagnosed based on the combination of bleeding and/or suppuration on probing, probing depths of more than or equal to 6 mm, and bone levels more than or equal to 3 mm apical to the intra-osseous part of the implant.[34]

RADIOGRAPHIC IMAGING IN PERI-IMPLANTITIS

The marginal bone around the implant crestal region serves as a crucial indicator of implant health. Measurement of the crestal bone level during initial surgery and subsequent radiographic evaluations are common methods to assess bone loss.[35] According to Froum and colleagues (2012), peri-implantitis severity was classified into 3 main categories based on probing depth and the amount of bone loss: early, moderate, and advanced. In the early stage, bone loss is less than or equal to 25% of the implant length, in the moderate stage, it ranges from 25% to 50% of the implant length, and in the advanced stage, bone loss exceeds 50% of the implant length.[36] The shape of the peri-implant defect plays a crucial role in interventions aimed at stopping and managing peri-implantitis.[37] Various radiographic techniques are available to assess the success of dental implants.[38] IRs are currently considered the standard method for assessing the marginal bone level around implants, which serves as the key indicator of peri-implantitis.[34] Additionally, panoramic radiographs can also be used for diagnosing peri-implantitis.[26] While IRs are sufficient for displaying the superimposed interproximal bone level, they lack the capability to visualize the facial and lingual/palatal bone[39] (**Fig. 9**A and B). However, 3D radiographs such as CBCT, enable the evaluation of all 4 bony walls of the defect, are considered superior to the 2D radiographs.[35] Moreover, CBCT provides enhanced information by allowing the evaluation of buccal and lingual bone plates around implants in both vertical and horizontal dimensions[40] (**Fig. 10**A–C). A study by Ritter and colleagues (2017) evaluated the accuracy of 3D CBCT and IRs in visualizing peri-implant bone when compared to histology. The study indicated that both CBCT and IR showed similar results in assessing medial and distal bone levels. However, CBCT proved to be superior in evaluating the oral and buccal bone, though with some limitations.[40] To comprehensively evaluate peri-implant bone dimensions, cross-sectional imaging becomes imperative. Conversely, while CBCT provides 3D images of peri-implant tissues; nonetheless, artifacts from metallic restorations and implants limit image quality and interpretation, particularly in cases with thin bone or potential fenestration/dehiscence.[41]

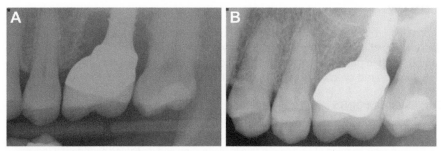

Fig. 9. (*A*) Periapical image for a tissue-level implant showing vertical bone loss on the mesial and distal aspects up to the second thread. (*B*) Six-months postoperative image showing significant bone regeneration following a regenerative procedure.

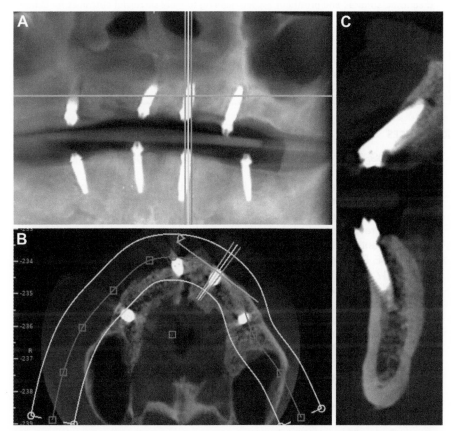

Fig. 10. Follow-up CBCT study for a case of full-arch implant restoration. (*A*) CBCT-reformatted panoramic image. (*B*) Axial view. (*C*) Cross-sectional views show bone loss on the facial aspect of dental implants.

SUMMARY

In conclusion, 2D and 3D radiographic imaging are valuable tool for periodontal and peri-implant disease management. It provides detailed information that can significantly enhance patient care and treatment outcomes. However, its use should be judicious and based on clinical indications to maximize benefits and minimize risks.

CLINICS CARE POINTS

- Radiographic imaging plays a crucial role in diagnosing and managing periodontal diseases. Two-dimensional (2D) radiographs, including bitewing, periapical, and panoramic images are commonly used. However, they have certain limitations, such as overlapping structures and potential underestimation of bone defects. To overcome these limitations, 3-dimensional imaging techniques, such as cone beam computed tomography (CBCT), have been introduced. CBCT offers high-resolution and detailed views. CBCT is particularly valuable in cases with extensive bone loss and furcation involvement.

- Radiographic examination is fundamental for planning and evaluating implant sites. While panoramic and intraoral periapical radiographs can provide valuable information, CBCT is considered superior for complex cases. It also facilitates proper coordination between diagnostic, surgical, and prosthetic aspects, leading to more successful outcomes for dental implant treatment.

- In the context of peri-implantitis, radiographic evaluation of the crestal bone level is crucial. Intraoral radiographs are commonly used for this purpose, but they may not fully visualize the facial and lingual/palatal bone. CBCT, provides a comprehensive evaluation of all bony walls of the defect and allows for better assessment of the buccal and lingual bone plates around implants in both vertical and horizontal dimensions.

REFERENCES

1. Gasner NS, Schure RS. In: Periodontal Disease. Treasure Island, FL: StatPearls Publishing; 2023.
2. Eke PI, Dye B, Wei L, et al, CDC Periodontal Disease Surveillance workgroup: James Beck University of North Carolina, Chapel Hill, USA, Gordon Douglass Past President, American Academy of Periodontology, Roy Page University of Washin. Prevalence of periodontitis in adults in the United States: 2009 and 2010. J Dent Res 2012;91(10):914–20.
3. Kinane DF, Stathopoulou PG, Papapanou PN. Periodontal diseases. Nat Rev Dis Prim 2017;3(1):1–14.
4. Korostoff J, Aratsu A, Kasten B, et al. Radiologic assessment of the periodontal patient. Dental Clinics 2016;60(1):91–104.
5. Scarfe WC, Azevedo B, Pinheiro LR, et al. The emerging role of maxillofacial radiology in the diagnosis and management of patients with complex periodontitis. Periodontology 2000 2017;74(1):116–39.
6. Tugnait A, Clerehugh V, Hirschmann P. The usefulness of radiographs in diagnosis and management of periodontal diseases: a review. J Dent 2000;28(4):219–26.
7. de Faria Vasconcelos K, Evangelista K, Rodrigues C, et al. Detection of periodontal bone loss using cone beam CT and intraoral radiography. Dentomaxillofacial Radiol 2012;41(1):64–9.
8. Misch KA, Yi ES, Sarment DP. Accuracy of cone beam computed tomography for periodontal defect measurements. J Periodontol 2006;77(7):1261–6.

9. Eickholz P, Kim T-S, Benn DK, et al. Validity of radiographic measurement of inter-proximal bone loss. Oral Surg Oral Med Oral Pathol Oral Radiol Endod 1998; 85(1):99–106.

10. Du Bois A, Kardachi B, Bartold P. Is there a role for the use of volumetric cone beam computed tomography in periodontics? Aust Dent J 2012;57:103–8.

11. Walter C, Kaner D, Berndt DC, et al. Three-dimensional imaging as a pre-operative tool in decision making for furcation surgery. J Clin Periodontol 2009;36(3): 250–7.

12. Acar B, Kamburoğlu K. Use of cone beam computed tomography in periodontology. World J Radiol 2014;6(5):139.

13. Mengel R, Candir M, Shiratori K, et al. Digital volume tomography in the diagnosis of periodontal defects: an in vitro study on native pig and human mandibles. J Periodontol 2005;76(5):665–73.

14. Noujeim M, Prihoda T, Langlais R, et al. Evaluation of high-resolution cone beam computed tomography in the detection of simulated interradicular bone lesions. Dentomaxillofacial Radiol 2009;38(3):156–62.

15. Braun X, Ritter L, Jervøe-Storm P-M, et al. Diagnostic accuracy of CBCT for periodontal lesions. Clin Oral Invest 2014;18:1229–36.

16. Leung CC, Palomo L, Griffith R, et al. Accuracy and reliability of cone-beam computed tomography for measuring alveolar bone height and detecting bony dehiscences and fenestrations. Am J Orthod Dentofacial Orthop 2010;137(4): S109–19.

17. McAllister BS, Eshraghi VT. Commentary: Cone-Beam Computed Tomography: An Essential Technology for Management of Complex Periodontal and Implant Cases. J Periodontol 2017;88(10):937–8.

18. Academy Of Osseointegration. 2010 Guidelines of the Academy of Osseointegration for the provision of dental implants and associated patient care. Int J Oral Maxillofac Implants 2010;25(3):620–7.

19. Harris D, Horner K, Gröndahl K, et al. EAO guidelines for the use of diagnostic imaging in implant dentistry 2011. A consensus workshop organized by the European Association for Osseointegration at the Medical University of Warsaw. Clin Oral Implants Res 2012;23(11):1243–53.

20. Benavides E, Rios HF, Ganz SD, et al. Use of cone beam computed tomography in implant dentistry: the International Congress of Oral Implantologists consensus report. Implant Dent 2012;21(2):78–86.

21. White SC, Scarfe WC, Schulze RK, et al. The Image Gently in Dentistry campaign: promotion of responsible use of maxillofacial radiology in dentistry for children. Oral Surgery, Oral Medicine, Oral Pathology and Oral Radiology 2014;118(3): 257–61.

22. Bornstein MM, Scarfe WC, Vaughn VM, et al. Cone beam computed tomography in implant dentistry: a systematic review focusing on guidelines, indications, and radiation dose risks. Int J Oral Maxillofac Implants 2014;29(Suppl):55–77.

23. Omami G, Al Yafi F. Should cone beam computed tomography be routinely obtained in implant planning? Dental Clinics 2019;63(3):363–79.

24. Rios HF, Borgnakke WS, Benavides E. The use of cone-beam computed tomography in management of patients requiring dental implants: an American Academy of Periodontology best evidence review. J Periodontol 2017;88(10):946–59.

25. Fokas G, Vaughn VM, Scarfe WC, et al. Accuracy of linear measurements on CBCT images related to presurgical implant treatment planning: A systematic review. Clin Oral Implants Res 2018;29:393–415.

26. Ramanauskaite A, Juodzbalys G. Diagnostic principles of peri-implantitis: a systematic review and guidelines for peri-implantitis diagnosis proposal. J Oral Maxillofac Res 2016;7(3):8.

27. Ismail AY, Shaddox LM, Santamaria MP, Al Sabbagh M, Peri-implantitis. A Review to Simplify a Mystifying Disease. Med Res Arch 2022;10(10).

28. Lang NP, Berglundh T, HeitzMayfield LJ, et al. Consensus statements and recommended clinical procedures regarding implant survival and complications. Int J Oral Maxillofac Implants 2004;19(Suppl):150–4.

29. Berglundh T, Persson L, Klinge B. A systematic review of the incidence of biological and technical complications in implant dentistry reported in prospective longitudinal studies of at least 5 years. J Clin Periodontol 2002;29:197–212.

30. Monje A, Galindo-Moreno P, Tözüm TF, et al. Into the Paradigm of Local Factors as Contributors for Peri-implant Disease: Short Communication. Int J Oral Maxillofac Implants 2016;31(2):288–92.

31. Schwarz F, Derks J, Monje A, et al. Peri-implantitis. J Clin Periodontol 2018;45: S246–66.

32. Lindhe J, Meyle J, GDotEWo Periodontology. Peri-implant diseases: consensus report of the sixth European workshop on periodontology. J Clin Periodontol 2008;35:282–5.

33. Derks J, Schaller D, Hakansson J, et al. Peri-implantitis–onset and pattern of progression. J Clin Periodontol 2016;43(4):383–8.

34. Berglundh T, Armitage G, Araujo MG, et al. Peri-implant diseases and conditions: Consensus report of workgroup 4 of the 2017 World Workshop on the Classification of Periodontal and Peri-Implant Diseases and Conditions. J Periodontol 2018; 89:S313–8.

35. Misch CE, Perel ML, Wang H-L, et al. Implant success, survival, and failure: the International Congress of Oral Implantologists (ICOI) pisa consensus conference. Implant Dent 2008;17(1):5–15.

36. Froum SJ, Rosen PS. A proposed classification for peri-implantitis. Int J Periodontics Restor Dent 2012;32(5):533.

37. Macías Y, Gañán Y, Macías Y, et al. Diagnostic Accuracy of Cone Beam Computed Tomography in Identifying Peri-implantitis–Like Bone Defects Ex Vivo. Int J Periodontics Restorative Dent 2021;41:e223–31.

38. Monsour P, Dudhia R. Implant radiography and radiology. Aust Dent J 2008;53: S11–25.

39. Monje A, Pons R, Insua A, et al. Morphology and severity of peri-implantitis bone defects. Clin Implant Dent Relat Res 2019;21(4):635–43.

40. Ritter L, Elger M, Rothamel D, et al. Accuracy of peri-implant bone evaluation using cone beam CT, digital intra-oral radiographs and histology. Dentomaxillofacial Radiol 2014;43(6):20130088.

41. de-Azevedo-Vaz SL, Peyneau PD, Ramirez-Sotelo LR, et al. Efficacy of a cone beam computed tomography metal artifact reduction algorithm for the detection of peri-implant fenestrations and dehiscences. Oral surgery, oral medicine, oral pathology and oral radiology 2016;121(5):550–6.

Inflammatory Lesions of the Jaws

Galal Omami, BDS, MSc, MDentSc, FRCD(C), Dip. ABOMR[a,*],
Richard H. Wiggins III, MD, CIIP, FSIIM[b]

KEYWORDS

- Periapical diseases • Osteomyelitis • Osteoradionecrosis
- Medication-related osteonecrosis

KEY POINTS

- The differential diagnosis of inflammatory jaw lesions remains broad and presents a diagnostic challenge to the practicing clinician.
- The imaging characteristics of inflammatory lesions evolve with disease chronicity.
- A strong knowledge of the clinical and radiographic features of inflammatory diseases is necessary to achieve a final diagnosis or at least narrow the differential considerations and lend confidence to clinical decision-making.
- An approach focusing on the spatial anatomy of the neck allows for accurate localization of infections involving the deep neck and helps determine the potential routes of spread of disease.

INTRODUCTION

Inflammatory lesions are the most common pathologic condition affecting the jaws, and they usually occur as sequelae of caries and periodontal disease. When the tooth has a necrotic pulp or a failing endodontic treatment and the inflammatory response is contained to the vicinity of the root apex, the condition is called a periapical inflammatory lesion (apical periodontitis). When the inflammation spreads into the bone marrow spaces, it is called osteomyelitis. Another source of inflammatory bone lesions is extension of inflammation from the gingival tissues into the underlying bone; this condition includes marginal periodontitis and pericoronitis. Apical periodontitis affects apical periodontal tissues, whereas marginal periodontitis affects coronal periodontal tissues. Osteonecrosis of jawbones is another inflammatory condition of bone that may result as a complication of radiotherapy to the head and neck or bisphosphonate

[a] Division of Oral Diagnosis, Oral Medicine, and Oral Radiology, Department of Oral Health Practice, University of Kentucky College of Dentistry, 770 Rose Street, MN320, Lexington, KY 40536, USA; [b] Department of Radiology and Imaging Sciences, University of Utah Health Sciences Center, 30 North 1900 East, Room 1A071, Salt Lake City, UT 84132, USA
* Corresponding author.
E-mail address: galal.omami@uky.edu

Dent Clin N Am 68 (2024) 259–276
https://doi.org/10.1016/j.cden.2023.09.003
0011-8532/24/© 2023 Elsevier Inc. All rights reserved.

therapy. This article provides an overview of the imaging appearance of inflammatory lesions of the jaws. Imaging of periodontal disease is discussed in A. Ismail & F. Al-Yafi, "The Role of Radiographic Imaging in the Diagnosis and Management of Periodontal and Peri-Implant Diseases", in this issue.

PERIAPICAL INFLAMMATORY LESIONS
Definition and Clinical Features

A periapical inflammatory lesion is a local response of the tissues around the apex of a tooth root that occurs as a result of pulpal necrosis secondary to caries or trauma. Periapical tissues consist of cementum, periodontal ligament, and alveolar bone. Histologically, the periapical inflammatory lesion may represent a periapical abscess (acute apical periodontitis) or a periapical granuloma (chronic apical periodontitis). Abscesses can transform into granulomas (and vice versa) without significant change in their radiographic appearance. Periapical inflammatory lesions are designated as symptomatic or asymptomatic based on their clinical presentations. If untreated, apical periodontitis may result in (1) periapical cyst formation, (2) abscess formation with a draining sinus tract, (3) development of facial cellulitis, or (4) development of osteomyelitis.

Imaging Features

The imaging features of periapical inflammatory lesions can range from no changes very early in their course to widening of the apical periodontal ligament space and effacement of the lamina dura to a mixture of rarefaction and sclerosis of periapical bone (**Fig. 1**A–D). When most of the lesion consists of sclerotic (radiopaque) changes, the term sclerosing osteitis is used. The periphery of sclerosing osteitis usually is ill-defined and blends gradually with surrounding trabeculae. With long-standing periapical inflammatory lesions, root resorption may occur, and cortical boundaries may be destroyed. These lesions can produce mucoperiosteal thickening in the adjacent floor of the maxillary sinus (**Fig. 2**A and B).

The differential diagnosis of periapical inflammatory lesions includes other radiolucent and sclerotic lesions that can exist at the root apex. These include periapical cemento-osseous dysplasia and idiopathic osteosclerosis (dense bone island). These conditions often cannot be distinguished from a periapical inflammatory lesion by radiographic findings alone; thus, the final diagnosis must rely on the clinical examination, including vitality testing of the involved tooth. Mature periapical cemento-osseous dysplasia can be differentiated from sclerosing osteitis by the presence of a thin radiolucent periphery. Also, periapical cemento-osseous dysplasia is often multifocal and predominantly involves the periapical region of the mandibular anterior teeth. Finally, external root resorption is more common with inflammatory lesions than with periapical cemento-osseous dysplasia. When idiopathic osteosclerosis is centered on the root apex, it may mimic periapical sclerosing osteitis. However, in idiopathic osteosclerosis, the periodontal membrane space around the apex of the tooth has a normal uniform width. In addition, the periphery of idiopathic osteosclerosis is usually well defined and does not blend in with surrounding bone.[1]

PERICORONITIS
Definition and Clinical Features

Pericoronitis is inflammation of the soft tissues surrounding the crown of a partially erupted tooth, most often a mandibular third molar. This condition usually occurs in young adults. The inflammatory process arises when food and bacterial debris become entrapped under the soft tissue flap covering the crown. Predisposing factors

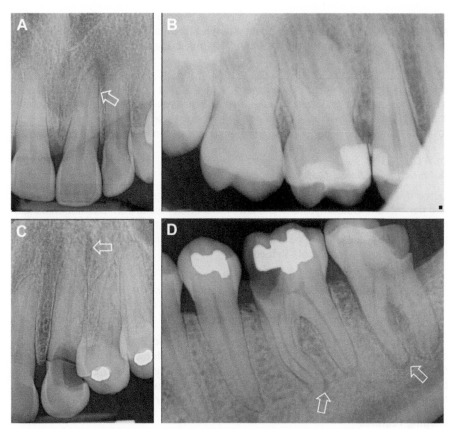

Fig. 1. Examples of periapical inflammatory lesions. Periapical inflammatory lesions (*arrows*) associated with a maxillary central incisor (*A*), maxillary first molar (*B*), maxillary canine (*C*), and mandibular first molar (*D*). Note the apical root resorption and widening of the pulp space (*A*). Also, note the gradual widening of the periodontal ligament space characteristic of an inflammatory lesion (*A, arrow*). The lesion is located along the root surface because of accessory canal (*C, arrow*). (*D*) Periapical sclerosing osteitis related to the first and second molars; note the associated widening of the periodontal ligament space (*arrows*).

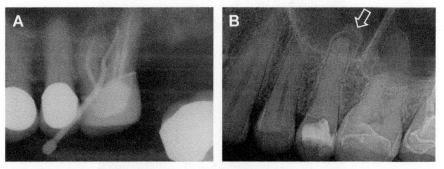

Fig. 2. Periapical inflammatory lesions. (*A*) Determining the source of the infection by threading a gutta-percha point through the sinus tract. (*B*) Periosteal reaction arises from a periapical inflammatory lesion on the second premolar (*arrow*). Also, note the calcification of the pulp canal.

include occlusal trauma, stress, and upper respiratory infection. Common clinical symptoms include pain, swelling, foul taste, and trismus. Systemic symptoms, such as fever, lymphadenopathy, and malaise, also may be noted.

Imaging Features

Because pericoronitis arises in soft tissues, in most cases no radiographic changes are seen. However, if the underlying bone is involved, features of osteitis or even osteomyelitis may develop, including enlargement of the follicular space of the involved tooth, sclerosis and rarefaction of surrounding bone, and periosteal new bone formation (**Fig. 3**).

OSTEOMYELITIS
Definition and Clinical Features

Osteomyelitis is inflammation of the entire bone including the marrow spaces, cortex, and periosteum. Osteomyelitis of the jaws most often results from odontogenic infections, extraction wounds, compound fractures, and radiation therapy. The disease has a strong male predilection. The mandible is affected much more often than the maxilla; this is most likely because of the following:

- The mandible is less vascular than the maxilla.
- Confinement of infections within the mandible because the cortical plates are thicker and denser.
- The mandible is a more common site for fracture.[2]

Patients with acute osteomyelitis experience a rapid onset of severe pain and swelling of the affected area. Fever, malaise, leukocytosis, and lymphadenopathy may be present. The associated tooth may demonstrate increased mobility and sensitivity to percussion. Purulent discharge also may be present. When the third division of the trigeminal nerve is involved, paresthesia of the lower lip may occur.

Imaging Features

No radiographic findings may be present in the acute phase of the disease, although there may be a slight decrease in the bone density, with blurring of the existing

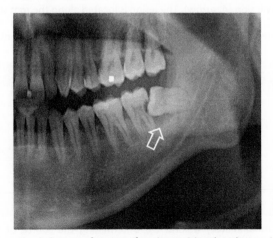

Fig. 3. Cropped panoramic image of a case of pericoronitis related to an impacted mandibular third molar. Note the changes of sclerosis and rarefaction of surrounding bone (*arrow*). Also note the carious/resorptive lesion on the distal aspect of the second molar.

trabeculae. As the disease progresses, bone resorption becomes more profound, resulting in a single or multiple irregular lytic areas with poorly defined margins. This pattern sometimes takes the form of moth-eaten bone. These changes are progressive and lead to fragmentation or sequestration of the cortex (**Figs. 4**A–C and **5**A–C). Diffuse sclerosing osteomyelitis is a chronic form of osteomyelitis with a prominent sclerotic response. Periosteal new bone formation may be seen in response to subperiosteal spread of the infection. This proliferation is more common in young patients and presents as single or multiple layers of bone that roughly parallel each other and the underlying cortical surface, resulting in an onion-skin appearance (**Fig. 6**A–C).[3]

Because acute osteomyelitis is often accompanied by extension of infection into the adjacent spaces, a contrast-enhanced computed tomography (CT) study is usually performed at this stage. The images should be obtained using both bone and soft-tissue algorithm. CT findings include a mixture of sclerosis and rarefaction, sequestrum formation, periosteal bone reaction, pathologic fracture, fistulous tracts,

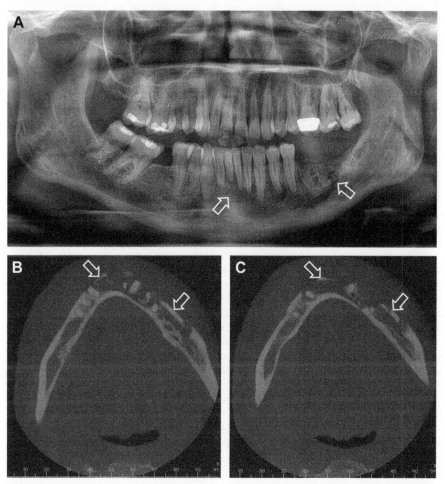

Fig. 4. Osteomyelitis of the mandible. (*A*) Panoramic view shows a mixed pattern of osteolysis and sclerosis in the left mandible (*arrows*). (*B* and *C*) Axial cone-beam CT images revealing multiple sequestra as detached segments of outer cortical bone (*arrows*).

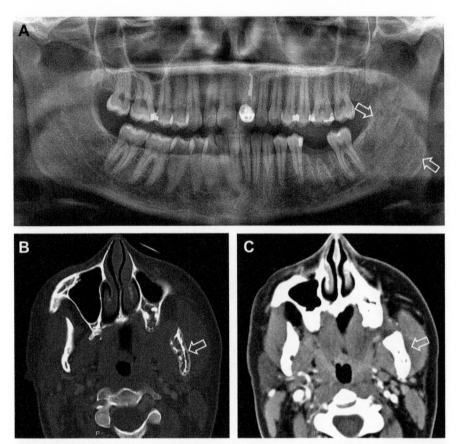

Fig. 5. Osteomyelitis of the mandible with masticator space infection. (*A*) Panoramic image shows lytic, "moth-eaten" destruction involving the left ramus (*arrow*). (*B*) Axial CT image displayed in bone window reveals permeative changes. Note the laminated periosteal reaction along the cortices (*arrow*). (*C*) Axial contrast-enhanced CT image displayed in soft-tissue window shows an early abscess in the left masticator space (focal low density, *arrow*) with swelling of the masseter muscle.

abscess formation, and cellulitis (**Table 1**). MR imaging can detect early-stage osteomyelitis before bone changes are evident on plain radiographs.[4] Inflammatory changes involving the bone marrow and soft tissues demonstrate high signal intensity on T2-weighted and STIR (short tau inversion recovery) images, low signal intensity on T1-weighted images, and enhancement after administration of intravenous contrast material (gadolinium).[4] Nuclear scintigraphy also plays a role in early diagnosis of osteomyelitis as technetium bone scan shows increased metabolism in the affected areas.[5]

The acute phase of osteomyelitis may yield a radiologic picture similar to malignant neoplasia. Careful examination typically reveals an apparent cause for osteomyelitis. In addition, osteomyelitis usually causes a reactive peripheral sclerosis, whereas malignant lesions do not.

Chronic osteomyelitis most often results in an increase in density and size of the jaw, giving a similar appearance to fibrous dysplasia. The size increase in osteomyelitis is due to the new bone laid down by the periosteum on the outer cortical

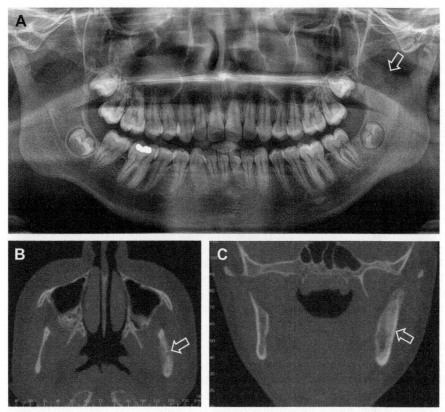

Fig. 6. Osteomyelitis with proliferative periostitis. (*A*) Panoramic radiograph shows an increase in density of the left mandibular ramus compared with the right side. Note the periosteal bone formation along the coronoid notch (*arrow*). Axial (*B*) and coronal (*C*) cone-beam CT images show an increase in density and size of the mandible. Note the multiple layers of new bone on the outer cortical plates of the mandible (*arrows*).

Table 1 Imaging findings of osteomyelitis	
Imaging Modality	**Findings**
Plain films/CBCT/CT	• Combination of bone sclerosis and bone destruction • Sequestrum • Periosteal new bone formation • Pathologic fracture • Cortical bone fistulae, abscess formation • Fasciitis, myositis, cellulitis
MR imaging	• Decrease in T1 signal intensity due to replacement of marrow fat by inflammation. • Increase in T2 signal intensity related to edema. • Contrast enhancement due to blood tissue barrier disruption.
Bone scintigraphy	• Increased radionuclide uptake "hot spot" reflecting hypermetabolic activity.

Abbreviations: CBCT, cone-beam computed tomography; CT, computed tomography.

surface. In contrast, the bone expansion associated with fibrous dysplasia is caused by replacement of the existing trabeculae by innumerable tiny trabeculae while thinning and displacing the outer cortex.[6] Bone sequestra are not seen in fibrous dysplasia. Osteosarcoma may produce a similar pattern and cause expansion, but it may stimulate a periosteal reaction that usually takes the form of "sunray" spiculation.

OSTEORADIONECROSIS
Definition and Clinical Features

Osteoradionecrosis is a pathologic condition of bone that results as a complication of radiation therapy for head and neck malignancy. Therapeutic radiation can damage the cellular elements of bone, and this can result in tissue hypocellularity, hypovascularity, and hypoxia. Bone healing capacity is also reduced, and necrosis may occur after bacterial invasion or surgical manipulation. The risk of osteoradionecrosis increases with the radiation dose absorbed by the bone, especially for those receiving more than 60 Gy.[7] The risk is also greater in patients with poor oral hygiene or ill-fitting dentures. The condition may develop at any time after the delivery of radiation therapy. The frequency of osteoradionecrosis is higher in the mandible and the posterior areas. The clinical hallmarks of osteoradionecrosis include intractable pain, surface ulceration, fistula formation, and bone exposure and sequestration. Progression of the condition may lead to a pathologic fracture. Histologically, necrotic bone demonstrates the loss of osteocytes from their lacunae.

Imaging Features

Osteoradionecrosis appears on imaging as foci of bone rarefaction and sclerosis (**Figs. 7**A, B and **8**). It often demonstrates skip lesions consisting of areas of destroyed cortex alternating with segments of spared cortex or sequestra, giving a "dot-dash" appearance (**Fig. 8**A–C). Periosteal bone reaction is uncommon. Distinction between osteoradionecrosis and recurrent malignancy can be difficult; however, the presence of bone sclerosis and the alternating areas of destroyed and spared cortex are characteristics of osteoradionecrosis and should distinguish it from tumor recurrence. Although uncommon, intraosseous gas is a useful CT feature to suggest osteoradionecrosis over recurrent tumor.[8] Bone scintigraphy using technetium-99m sestamibi or

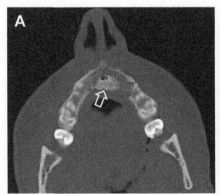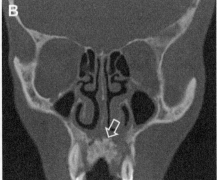

Fig. 7. Osteoradionecrosis of the maxilla. Axial (A) and coronal (B) CT images in bone window show osteolytic and sclerotic changes in the anterior maxilla (arrows). Note the lack of periosteal bone reaction. This patient had radiation therapy for a sinonasal lymphoma.

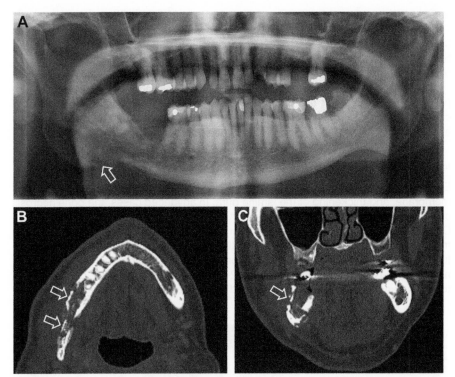

Fig. 8. Osteoradionecrosis of the mandible. (*A*) Panoramic image shows a patchy, "moth-eaten" pattern of bone destruction involving the right body of the mandible. A pathologic fracture is also present (*arrow*). Axial (*B*) and coronal (*C*) CT images show cortical fragmentation. Note the skip lesions of the buccal cortex; areas of destroyed cortex interspersed with segments of spared cortex or sequestra (*arrows*). There is minimal periosteal bone reaction. This patient had radiation therapy for a tongue carcinoma.

thallium-201 may be helpful in differentiating osteoradionecrosis from recurrent cancer.[9,10] Areas of necrotic bone demonstrate decreased tracer uptake, as opposed to viable tumor that shows intense uptake. Differentiation from osteomyelitis should not be difficult because of the history of radiation therapy.

MEDICATION-RELATED OSTEONECROSIS OF THE JAWS
Definition and Clinical Features

Bisphosphonates and other antiresorptive agents (eg, denosumab) are commonly used to reduce bone resorption and pain in patients with multiple myeloma, skeletal metastasis, Paget's disease of bone, or osteoporosis. These drugs are also effective in treating hypercalcemia of malignancy. They inhibit osteoclastic activity and possibly interfere with angiogenesis. The initial association between bisphosphonates use and subsequent development of osteonecrosis of the jaw was documented in 2003.[11] Since then, many cases of bisphosphonate-related osteonecrosis of the jaw have been reported. The current preferred term for this condition is medication-related osteonecrosis of the jaw (MRONJ) or antiresorptive agent-related osteonecrosis of the jaw.[12] The clinical criteria for diagnosing MRONJ include all the following elements: (1) current or previous history of antiresorptive therapy; (2) exposed bone that has persisted for more than 8 weeks; and (3) no history of radiation therapy to the jaws.[13] The risk for MRONJ in patients with osteoporosis and cancer has been reported as 0.06% and 1.47%, respectively.[14] The pathogenesis of MRONJ remains unclear, but it seems to result from a complex interplay of bone metabolism, infection, trauma, hypovascularity, immunity, and genetics.

Affected patients have an area of exposed necrotic bone that may or may not be painful. The precipitating event is often an invasive dental procedure such as tooth extraction. However, cases related to denture trauma and spontaneous cases have also occurred. The mandible is affected three times more often than the maxilla.

Imaging Features

Early in the disease, there may be diffuse bone sclerosis, widening of the periodontal membrane, and thickening of the lamina dura. In advanced cases, the bone necrosis creates irregular, "moth-eaten" bone destruction with or without sequestra (**Figs. 9**A–C and **10**A and B). There may be lucent tunneling along the cortex leading to cortical fragmentation. Periosteal new bone formation is seen occasionally.[15] Pathologic fractures may occur as a sequela of destruction of the mandibular bone. On MR imaging, necrotic bone has low T1-weighted and T2-weighted signal intensities corresponding to low water content, hypovascularity, and hypocellularity.[16]

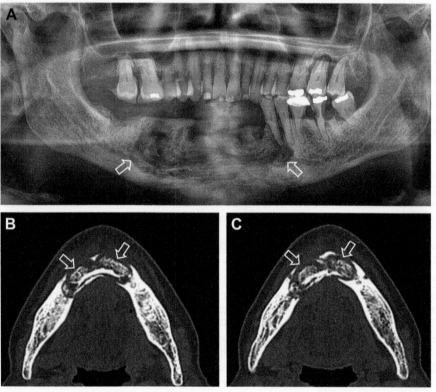

Fig. 9. Medication-related osteonecrosis of the jaws. (*A*) Panoramic view shows extensive bone destruction and sclerosis involving the anterior segment of the mandible (*arrows*). (*B, C*) Axial CT images reveal cortical fragmentation and sequestrum formation (*arrows*).

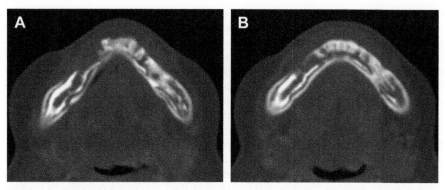

Fig. 10. Medication-related osteonecrosis of the jaws. (*A, B*) Axial CT images show fragmentation and sequestrum formation affecting the entire mandible. The sequestration is so extensive that it suggests a "bone-within-bone" appearance.

DEEP FACE AND NECK INFECTIONS
Fasciae and Spaces of the Neck

Familiarity with the fasciae and spaces of the neck is essential for proper evaluation of patients with deep face and neck infections. These fasciae define spaces that limit to a certain degree the spread of infections and tumors. The fasciae of the neck are traditionally classified into two major divisions: superficial and deep. The superficial

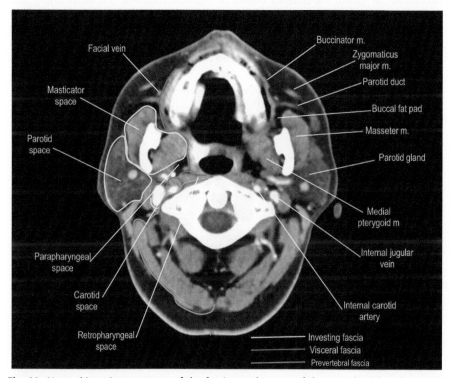

Fig. 11. Normal imaging anatomy of the fasciae and spaces of the suprahyoid neck on axial contrast-enhanced CT image.

cervical fascia consists of the subcutaneous tissues and contains the platysma muscle. The deep cervical fascia is classically subdivided into three separate layers: (1) the superficial (investing) layer of deep cervical fascia, (2) the middle (visceral or buccopharyngeal) layer of deep cervical fascia, and (3) the deep (prevertebral) layer of deep cervical fascia (**Fig. 11**). The investing fascia is a well-defined, thick sheet of fibrous tissue that encircles the neck, surrounding the sternocleidomastoid and trapezius muscles. The visceral (buccopharyngeal) fascia envelops the visceral structures of the neck (pharynx, larynx, trachea, esophagus, and thyroid and parathyroid glands). The prevertebral fascia surrounds the spine and paraspinal muscles. The investing fascia splits to enclose the muscles of mastication (masseter, pterygoid muscles, and temporalis tendon) and the ramus of the mandible before attaching to the zygomatic arch, thereby forming the masticator space (see **Fig. 11**). The fascia splits once again to enclose the zygomatic arch and then continues cranially to contain the temporalis muscle. The investing fascia also splits to enclose the parotid and submandibular glands. In radiological literature, the submandibular space refers to the entire area superficial (inferior) to the mylohyoid muscle down to the investing fascia as it extends from the hyoid bone to the mandible (**Fig. 12**). The sublingual space is the area deep (superior) to the mylohyoid muscle up to the mucosa of the floor of the mouth on each side of the root of the tongue, creating a "horseshoe" shape in the axial plane. The submandibular and sublingual spaces are continuous posteriorly around the posterior free margin of the mylohyoid muscle at the glosso-mylohyoid gap. There is also free communication between the right and left sides of these spaces. The contents of the submandibular space include the superficial lobe of the submandibular gland, the anterior bellies of digastric muscles, the facial artery and vein, lymph nodes, and fat. The sublingual space contains the deep lobe and hilum of the submandibular gland, the submandibular duct (Wharton's duct), the sublingual gland, the hyoglossus muscle, the lingual artery and vein, the lingual and hypoglossal nerves, and fat. The buccal space is bounded by the superior and inferior attachments

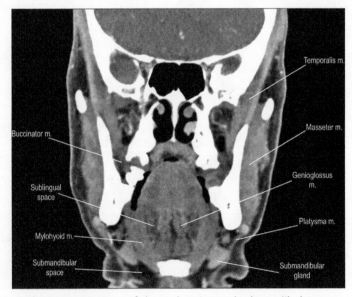

Fig. 12. Normal imaging anatomy of the oral region and submandibular space on coronal contrast-enhanced CT image.

of the buccinator muscle. It lies superficial to buccinator muscle, deep to the zygomaticus major muscle, and anterior to the masseter muscle. It contains the buccal fat pad, the parotid duct (Stensen's duct), the facial artery and vein, and the buccal division of the facial nerve. The parapharyngeal space is a fat-filled space on either side of the suprahyoid neck. It is formed by the superficial and middle layers of deep cervical fascia. It lies just lateral to the pharyngeal mucosal space, medial to the parotid space, and medial and posterior to the masticator space (see **Fig. 11**). The parapharyngeal space communicates freely with the submandibular and sublingual spaces inferiorly.

Imaging of Deep Face and Neck Infections

Infections within the oral region and adjacent spaces most commonly result from either dental infections or manipulation or from stones within the salivary gland ductal

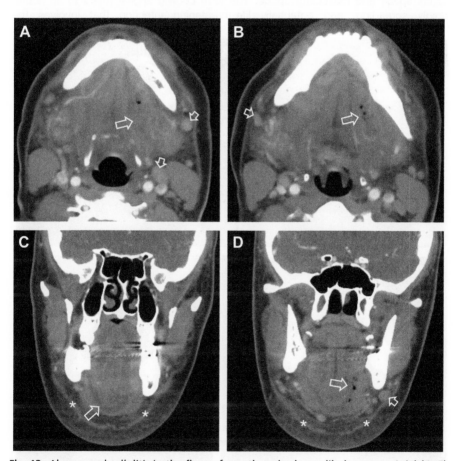

Fig. 13. Abscess and cellulitis in the floor of mouth and submandibular space. Axial (*A, B*) and coronal (*C, D*) contrast-enhanced CT images show diffuse inflammatory changes in the sublingual and submandibular spaces. Early abscess formation is seen in the floor of mouth (sublingual space) with gas collections (*long arrows*). Note other inflammatory changes including stranding of the subcutaneous fat suggestive of cellulitis, thickening of platysma muscle (*asterisks*), and multiple bilateral reactive lymph nodes (*short arrows*). Although this patient did not present with airway symptoms, the imaging appearance could be that of Ludwig angina.

systems. The mandibular molars are the most frequent cause of odontogenic infection.[4] It has been suggested the relationship of the root apices of the mandibular teeth to the attachment of the mylohyoid muscle may predict the pattern of spread of the infection. Unlike the roots of the mandibular first molar and premolars, the roots of the mandibular second and third molars extend below the mylohyoid muscle. As a result, infections arising from the mandibular first molar and premolars may preferentially involve the sublingual space, whereas infections arising from mandibular second and third molars may preferentially spread into the submandibular space.[17] In many cases, infections are multispatial, involving multiple contiguous spaces.[18] A submandibular space infection may spread into the sublingual space (and vice versa), the masticator space, the parapharyngeal space, and from there into the retropharyngeal space. Odontogenic infections of the maxillary molars may produce abscesses in the buccal space and masticator space. The term *Ludwig angina* refers to an acute, rapidly spreading, and potentially life-threatening infection that involves the

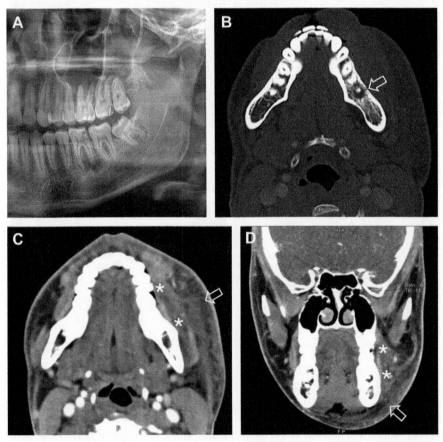

Fig. 14. Carious molar with periapical abscess and cellulitis. (*A*) Cropped panoramic image shows a periapical inflammatory lesion on the mandibular first molar. (*B*) Axial CT image in bone window demonstrates radiolucency around the mandibular first molar with perforation of the adjacent buccal cortex (*arrow*). Axial (*C*) and coronal (*D*) contrast-enhanced CT images in soft tissue window show buccinator myositis (*asterisks*) with diffuse stranding of the subcutaneous fat in the buccal and submandibular spaces (*arrows*) consistent with cellulitis.

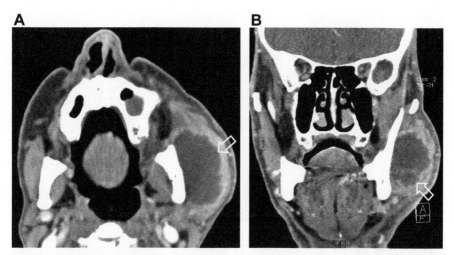

Fig. 15. Masticator space abscess. Axial (*A*) and coronal (*B*) contrast-enhanced CT images demonstrate a large, rim-enhancing, low-density lesion (*arrows*) in the left masticator space with surrounding cellulitis. This abscess was secondary to extraction of a carious mandibular third molar.

sublingual, submandibular, and submental spaces (**Fig. 13**A–D).[19] The infection causes firm induration of the floor of the mouth and elevation and posterior displacement of the tongue, which may lead to respiratory distress and toxic appearance. Affected patients present with diffuse swelling, oral pain, drooling, dysphagia, dysphonia, and stridor. Fever, chills, malaise, and leukocytosis may be present.[20]

Contrast-enhanced CT is the modality of choice for evaluation of oral cavity infections because of its superior ability to demonstrate both bone and soft tissue detail. The classic imaging manifestation of inflammation is cellulitis, which is seen as reticulation or stranding of the subcutaneous fat ("dirty fat") as a result of edema as well as the dilated venules and lymphatics, thickening and enhancement of the overlying skin

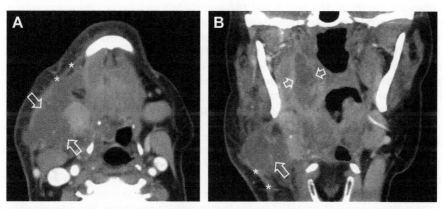

Fig. 16. Multispatial abscess after extraction of a carious mandibular third molar. Axial (*A*) and coronal (*B*) contrast-enhanced CT images show a large rim-enhancing low-attenuation collection within the submandibular space (*long arrows*), with extension into the parapharyngeal space (*short arrows*). There is thickening of the overlying skin, stranding of the subcutaneous fat, and thickening of the platysma (*asterisks*) as a result of inflammatory myositis.

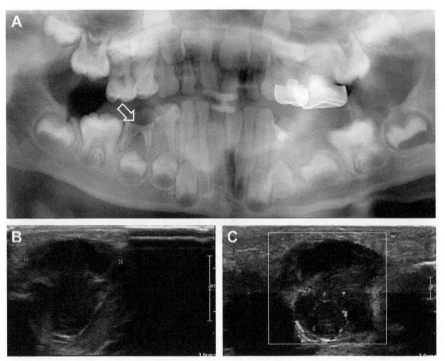

Fig. 17. Carious molar tooth with submandibular space abscess. (*A*) Panoramic image shows a periapical inflammatory lesion associated with the right mandibular primary second molar (*arrow*). (*B*) Sagittal ultrasonographic image shows a heterogenous, hypoechoic area representing abscess centered in the right submandibular space (calipers). (*C*) Transverse ultrasonographic image with color flow Doppler shows increased peripheral vascularity.

and adjacent muscles, and gas collections in the soft tissue (**Fig. 14**A–D). The presence of an abscess is seen as a localized area of low attenuation surrounded by an enhancing rim (**Figs. 15**A and B and **16**A and B). MR imaging or ultrasonography is recommended for pediatric patients and adults in whom the use of iodinated contrast is contraindicated.[17] On MR imaging, an abscess typically has hypointense signal on T1-weighted images, hyperintense signal on T2-weighted images, and peripheral rim enhancement following the administration of gadolinium. Reactive adenopathy involving the cervical lymph nodes may be visualized on MR and CT images (see **Fig. 13**). On ultrasonography, an abscess appears as a hypoechoic lesion with an increased peripheral blood flow on color Doppler imaging (**Fig. 17**A–C).

SUMMARY

The differential diagnosis of inflammatory jaw lesions remains broad and presents a diagnostic challenge to the practicing clinician. The radiologic analysis of these lesions may be approached by categorizing the lesion according to its anatomic location, periphery, internal aspect, and relationship to surrounding structures. The imaging characteristics of inflammatory lesions evolve with disease chronicity. A strong knowledge of the clinical and radiographic features of inflammatory diseases is necessary to achieve a final diagnosis or at least narrow the differential considerations and lend confidence to clinical decision-making. An approach focusing on the spatial anatomy of the neck allows for accurate localization of infections involving the deep neck and helps determine the potential routes of spread of disease.

DISCLOSURE

The authors declare that they have no conflict of interest.

REFERENCES

1. Lee Linda. Inflammatory disease. In: White S, Pharoah M, editors. Oral radiology: principles & interpretation. 7th edition. St Louis (MO): Elsevier; 2014. p. 314–33.
2. Baltensperger M, Eyrich G. Osteomyelitis of the jaws: definition and classification. In: Baltensperger M, Eyrich G, editors. Osteomyelitis of the jaws. Berlin, Heidelberg: Springer; 2009. p. 5–56.
3. Schuknecht B. Diagnostic imaging – conventional radiology, computed tomography and magnetic resonance imaging. In: Baltensperger M, Eyrich G, editors. Osteomyelitis of the jaws. Berlin, Heidelberg: Springer; 2009. p. 57–94.
4. Kaneda T, Minami M, Ozawa K, et al. Magnetic resonance imaging of osteomyelitis in the mandible: comparative study with other radiologic modalities. Oral Surg Oral Med Oral Pathol Oral Radiol Endod 1995;79:634–40.
5. Hardt N, Hofer B, Baltensperger M. Diagnostic imaging – scintigraphy. In: Baltensperger M, Eyrich G, editors. Osteomyelitis of the jaws. Berlin, Heidelberg: Springer; 2009. p. 95–111.
6. Petrikowski CG, Pharoah MJ, Lee L, et al. Radiographic differentiation of osteogenic sarcoma, osteomyelitis, and fibrous dysplasia of the jaws. Oral Surg Oral Med Oral Pathol Oral Radiol Endod 1995;80(6):744–50.
7. Mallya SM, Tetradis S. Imaging of radiation- and medication-related osteonecrosis. Radiol Clin North Am 2018;56(1):77–89.
8. Alhilali L, Reynolds AR, Fakhran S. Osteoradionecrosis after radiation therapy for head and neck cancer: differentiation from recurrent disease with CT and PET/CT imaging. AJNR Am J Neuroradiol 2014;35(7):1405–11.
9. Wang CH, Liang JA, Ding HJ, et al. Utility of TL-201 SPECT in clarifying false-positive FDG-PET findings due to osteoradionecrosis in head and neck cancer. Head Neck 2010;32(12):1648–54.
10. Tan AEH, Ng DCE. Differentiating osteoradionecrosis from nasopharyngeal carcinoma tumour recurrence using [99]Tcmsestamibi SPECT/CT. Br J Radiol 2011; 84(1005):172–5.
11. Marx RE. Pamidronate (Aredia) and zoledronate (Zometa) induced avascular necrosis of the jaws: a growing epidemic. J Oral Maxillofac Surg 2003;61(9): 1115–7.
12. Hellstein JW, Adler RA, Edwards B, et al. Managing the care of patients receiving antiresorptive therapy for prevention and treatment of osteoporosis: executive summary of recommendations from the American Dental Association Council on Scientific Affairs. J Am Dent Assoc 2011;142(11):1243–51.
13. Ruggiero SL, Dodson TB, Aghaloo T, et al. American Association of Oral and Maxillofacial Surgeons' position paper on medication-related osteonecrosis of the jaws-2022 Update. J Oral Maxillofac Surg 2022;80(5):920–43.
14. Ishimaru M, Ono S, Morita K, et al. Prevalence, incidence rate, and risk factors of medication-related osteonecrosis of the jaw in patients with osteoporosis and cancer: a nationwide population-based study in Japan. J Oral Maxillofac Surg 2022;80(4):714–27.

15. Baba A, Goto TK, Ojiri H, et al. CT imaging features of antiresorptive agent-related osteonecrosis of the jaw/medication-related osteonecrosis of the jaw. Dentomaxillofac Radiol 2018;47(4):20170323.

16. Bedogni A, Blandamura S, Lokmic Z, et al. Bisphosphonate-associated jawbone osteonecrosis: a correlation between imaging techniques and histopathology. Oral Surg Oral Med Oral Pathol Oral Radiol Endod 2008;105:358–64.

17. Forghani R, Smoker W, Curtin H. Pathology of the oral region. In: Som PM, Curtin HD, editors. Head and neck imaging. 5th edition. St. Louis, MO: Mosby; 2011. p. 1643–748.

18. Ariji Y, Gotoh M, Kimura Y, et al. Odontogenic infection pathway to the submandibular space: imaging assessment. Int J Oral Maxillofac Surg 2002;31:165–9.

19. Vieira F, Allen SM, Stocks RM, et al. Deep neck infection. Otolaryngol Clin North Am 2008;41:459–83.

20. Neville BW, Damm DD, Allen CM, et al. Pulpal and periapical disease. In: Neville BW, Damm DD, Allen CM, et al, editors. Oral and maxillofacial pathology. 3rd edition. Philadelphia, PA: Saunders; 2008. p. 120–53.

Cysts and Benign Odontogenic Tumors of the Jaws

Galal Omami, BDS, MSc, MDentSc, FRCD(C), Dip. ABOMR[a],*,
Melvyn Yeoh, MD, DMD[b]

KEYWORDS

- Jaw cysts • Odontogenic tumors • Cone-beam computed tomography
- Radiography

KEY POINTS

- Benign odontogenic lesions frequently occur in the jaws and appear radiographically as well-defined unilocular or multilocular radiolucent areas.
- The epicenter of odontogenic lesions is located above the inferior alveolar canal in the mandible and below the sinus floor in the maxilla.
- Odontogenic lesions are frequently associated with an impacted tooth, and the lesion's relationship to the tooth is an important differential diagnostic feature.
- Computed tomography imaging is especially useful to reveal regions of perforation of the expanded cortical plates.
- In most cases, microscopic examination of the specimen is necessary to establish a definitive diagnosis.

INTRODUCTION

A cyst is a pathologic cavity filled with fluid, lined by epithelium, and surrounded by a fibrous connective tissue wall. The classification proposed in this article divides the cysts of the jaws into odontogenic and nonodontogenic cysts. Odontogenic cysts are further subclassified as inflammatory and developmental in origin (**Box 1**). Non–epithelial-lined cysts (pseudocysts) are not discussed in this article.

Odontogenic tumors comprise a complex group of lesions that range from tumor-like malformations (hamartomas) to benign tumors to malignant carcinomas. These lesions are derived from remnants of the dental apparatus. Odontogenic tumors are classified into 3 basic groups: (1) tumors of odontogenic epithelium, composed only of odontogenic epithelium without odontogenic ectomesenchyme, (2) mixed odontogenic

[a] Division of Oral Diagnosis, Oral Medicine, and Oral Radiology, Department of Oral Health Practice, University of Kentucky College of Dentistry, 770 Rose Street, MN320, Lexington, KY 40536, USA; [b] Division of Oral and Maxillofacial Surgery, University of Kentucky College of Dentistry, 770 Rose Street, D-528, Lexington, KY 40536, USA
* Corresponding author.
E-mail address: galal.omami@uky.edu

Dent Clin N Am 68 (2024) 277–295
https://doi.org/10.1016/j.cden.2023.09.004
0011-8532/24/© 2023 Elsevier Inc. All rights reserved.

Box 1
Classifications of cysts of the jaws

I.Odontogenic
  A.Inflammatory
    Radicular cyst, apical, and lateral
    Residual radicular cyst
    Inflammatory collateral cyst
    Buccal bifurcation cyst (paradental cyst)
  B.Developmental
    Dentigerous cyst
    Odontogenic keratocyst
    Orthokeratinized odontogenic cyst
    Lateral periodontal cyst
    Glandular odontogenic cyst
    Calcifying odontogenic cyst

II.Nonodontogenic
    Nasopalatine duct cyst
    Nasolabial cyst
    Palatal cyst of the newborn

---

tumors, composed of odontogenic epithelium with odontogenic ectomesenchyme, and (3) tumors of odontogenic ectomesenchyme, composed essentially of odontogenic ectomesenchyme (**Box 2**).

Radicular Cyst

Definition and clinical features

Radicular cysts are the most common cysts of the jaws, representing 60% of all odontogenic cysts.[1] They originate from inflammatory proliferation of the epithelial rests of Malassez in the periodontal ligament as sequelae to periapical periodontitis following necrosis of the pulp. The epicenter of a radicular cyst is typically located at the apex of a nonvital tooth but it may also be located on the lateral aspect of a tooth root in relation to a lateral accessory canal (**Fig. 1**A, B and **2**). A radicular cyst that remains after removal of the offending tooth is termed a *residual cyst* (**Fig. 3**A, B). Rarely, an inflammatory cyst, termed an *inflammatory collateral cyst*, may develop in a deep periodontal pocket.[2]

Box 2
Classification of benign odontogenic tumors

I.Tumors of odontogenic epithelium
  A.Ameloblastoma (solid/multicystic, unicystic, and desmoplastic types)
  B.Adenomatoid odontogenic tumor
  C.Calcifying epithelial odontogenic tumor
  D.Squamous odontogenic tumor

II.Mixed odontogenic tumors
  A.Odontoma (complex and compound types)
  B.Ameloblastic fibroma
  C.Ameloblastic fibro-odontoma

III.Tumors of odontogenic ectomesenchyme
  A.Odontogenic myxoma
  B.Odontogenic fibroma
  C.Cementoblastoma

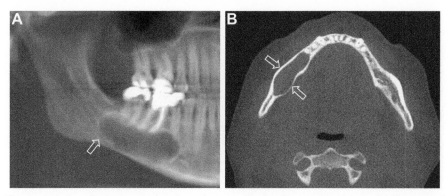

Fig. 1. Apical radicular cyst related to the mandibular first molar. Cropped reformatted panoramic (*A*) and (*B*) axial cone-beam CT images show a well-defined, elliptical, corticated radiolucency in the periapical areas of the mandibular second premolar and first and second molars. Note the epicenter is apical to the first molar. The cyst has caused thinning and expansion of the cortical plates (*arrows* in B) as well as inferior displacement of the mandibular canal (*arrow* in A).

Approximately 60% of radicular cysts occur in the maxilla, most often in the anterior region. Lesions usually produce no symptoms, unless secondary infection has occurred. Large lesions may cause swelling of the jaws. If the lesion perforates the outer cortex, the swelling may feel fluctuant. Needle aspiration often produces straw-colored fluid, although the cholesterol crystals present in the fluid may impart a shimmering gold color.[2]

Imaging features
Radicular cysts have well-defined and corticated periphery with a curved or circular outline. If a secondary infection is present, the cortex may be lost or altered into a thicker sclerotic border. The cyst often flattens out as it approaches cortical boundaries. The internal aspect of the lesion is usually radiolucent. Long-standing chronically inflamed cysts may exhibit dystrophic calcification appearing as sparsely scattered radiopaque foci. If the cyst is large enough, it may displace and resorb the adjacent teeth and cause smooth expansion and thinning of the outer cortical

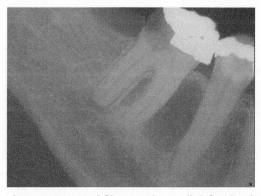

Fig. 2. Lateral radicular cyst. Periapical film reveals a well-defined radiolucency extending laterally from the mesial root of the first molar. The circular shape of the cyst is influenced by the adjacent roots.

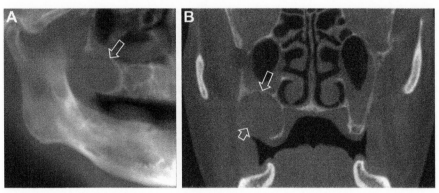

Fig. 3. Residual cyst in the maxilla. Cropped reformatted panoramic (*A*) and coronal (*B*) cone-beam CT images show a well-defined, expansile, radiolucent lesion in the posterior maxilla. Note the circular or "hydraulic" shape and the presence of a peripheral cortex. The lesion has caused elevation of the sinus floor (*long arrows*) and perforation of the buccal cortex (*short arrow*).

plates leaving a thin shell of bone. The cyst may elevate the floor of the maxillary antrum or depress the mandibular canal.[3]

Buccal Bifurcation Cyst

Definition and clinical features

The buccal bifurcation cyst (also referred to as a paradental cyst) is an inflammatory odontogenic cyst that characteristically develops on the buccal aspect of an erupting mandibular molar because of an inflammatory process in the periodontal pocket. Some of the involved teeth demonstrate buccal enamel extension from the cementoenamel junction toward the bifurcation region.[4] The patient may have a hard swelling on the buccal aspect of the involved tooth. Pain may occur when the cyst becomes secondarily infected. Periodontal examination usually reveals a deep probing defect in the buccal furcation of the affected molar.

Imaging features

Radiographs typically show a well-circumscribed unilocular radiolucency centered over the furcation area and surrounding the roots of the molar. The associated tooth is usually tilted so that the root apices may be displaced into the lingual mandibular cortex, a

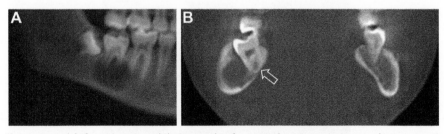

Fig. 4. Buccal bifurcation cyst. (*A*) Cropped reformatted panoramic image shows a cystic lesion on the roots of the mandibular second molar. The occlusal surface of the involved tooth has been tipped in relation to the first molar. (*B*) Coronal cone-beam CT image shows buccal expansion and displacement of the root tips of the second molar into the lingual cortical plate (*arrow*).

feature that is demonstrable on cross-sectional imaging (**Fig. 4**A and B).[3] The lesion may cause thinning and expansion of the buccal cortical plate. Periosteal reaction may occur on the buccal surface when the cyst becomes secondarily infected.

Dentigerous Cyst

Definition and clinical features

The dentigerous cyst is the most common type of developmental odontogenic cyst, accounting for about 18% of all odontogenic cysts.[1] It develops around the crown of an unerupted tooth by accumulation of fluid between the reduced enamel epithelium and the tooth crown. This cyst is most commonly seen in younger patients, with a peak prevalence in the second and third decades of life. There is a slight male predilection. Dentigerous cyst most often occurs in association with the mandibular third molars. Other frequently involved teeth include the maxillary canines, followed by the maxillary third molars and mandibular second premolars. Small lesions are typically asymptomatic and are discovered during routine dental examination. Larger lesions may cause painless swelling of the jaw.

Imaging features

Dentigerous cyst appears as a well-defined, smoothly curved, corticated, unilocular radiolucency surrounding the crown of an unerupted tooth and attached to its cementoenamel junction (**Fig. 5**A–C). An infected cyst may have noncorticated borders. As the cyst enlarges, it can cause expansion of the adjacent cortical plates of the involved jaw. Dentigerous cyst tends to displace and resorb adjacent teeth. The associated tooth is usually displaced in an apical direction, a finding that reinforces the impression that the epicenter of the lesion is coronal to the tooth. Large cysts in the mandible often displace the mandibular canal inferiorly. When the cyst develops in relation to the maxillary sinus, the sinus floor may be displaced as the lesion invaginates into the sinus cavity. A dentigerous cyst involving the sinus may spontaneously collapse and fill in with new bone (**Fig. 6**A and B). A small dentigerous cyst may be difficult, if not impossible, to distinguish from a hyperplastic follicle. However, for the lesion to be considered a dentigerous cyst, the size of the follicular space should exceed 5 mm.[3] Extremely large lesions may have undulating borders due to uneven expansion through the surrounding structures, resulting in an appearance similar to that of an odontogenic keratocyst (OKC) or ameloblastoma.[5] Rarely, a radicular cyst associated with a mandibular deciduous molar appears to be in a false dentigerous relationship with the erupting premolar, which has notched the cyst wall (**Fig. 7**).[6]

Odontogenic Keratocyst

Definition and clinical features

The most recent (fourth) edition of the World Health Organization Classification of Head and Neck Tumors has reclassified keratocystic odontogenic tumor as OKC.[7] These lesions are thought to originate from remnants of the dental lamina, and they account for 10% of all cystic lesions of the jaws. OKCs are seen in a wide age range, with a peak age of incidence in the second and third decades of life, and there is a slight male predominance. About 70% of lesions occur in the mandible, most often in the molar-ramus area. The lesion is often filled with yellow-white cheesy material (keratin). Although histologically benign, these lesions frequently exhibit locally aggressive behavior with a high recurrence rate. Multiple OKCs may be associated with nevoid basal cell carcinoma syndrome (Gorlin syndrome), an autosomal dominant disorder in which patients also develop multiple basal cell carcinomas, palmar and plantar pitting, dural calcification, and skeletal abnormalities.

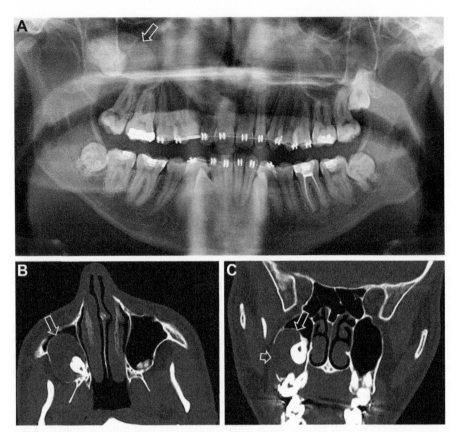

Fig. 5. Dentigerous cyst in the maxilla. (*A*) Panoramic film shows a well-defined, corticated, smooth, soft-tissue opacity associated with the maxillary right third molar, which has been displaced (*arrow*). Axial (*B*) and coronal (*C*) CT images show an expansile cystic lesion surrounding the crown of the third molar. Note the attachment of the cyst at the cementoenamel junction. The cyst elevates the sinus floor because it invaginates the antrum. The cortex represents the sinus floor bowing upward (*long arrow* in B and C). The lesion has caused erosion of the lateral antral wall (*short arrow* in C).

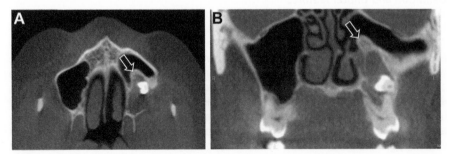

Fig. 6. Axial (*A*) and coronal (*B*) cone-beam CT images of a collapsing dentigerous cyst within the maxillary sinus. Note the reactive sclerotic bone along the cyst wall (*arrows*).

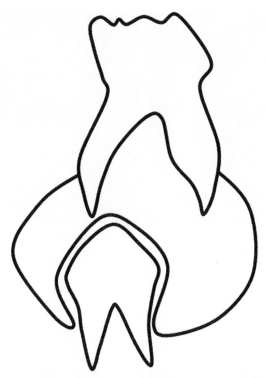

Fig. 7. Diagram illustrating the manner in which a radicular cyst associated with a deciduous molar may appear to be in a false pericoronal relationship with the erupting premolar.

Imaging features

Radiographically, the lesion manifests as a circumscribed unilocular or multilocular radiolucency with smooth or scalloped cortical margins (**Fig. 8**A and B and **9**A and B). Some cases are associated with an unerupted tooth. Small lesions can present as an interradicular radiolucency, resembling a lateral periodontal cyst.[8] An important diagnostic point is that this lesion tends to grow in an anteroposterior direction along the cancellous component of the mandible without causing significant expansion of the

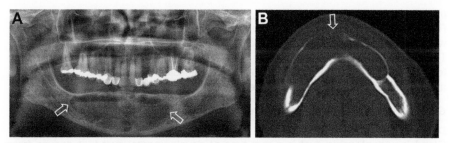

Fig. 8. Odontogenic keratocyst of the mandible. (*A*) Panoramic radiograph shows a well-circumscribed radiolucency in the mandibular symphysis and body on the right side (*arrows*). Note the scalloping of the endosteal surface of the inferior border, giving the false impression of internal septa. (*B*) Axial CT (bone window setting) shows expansion and erosion of the buccal cortical plate (*arrow*) and, to a lesser degree, the lingual plate.

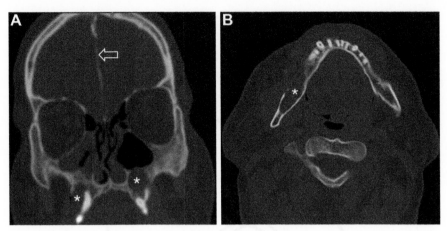

Fig. 9. Nevoid basal cell carcinoma (Gorlin) syndrome. Coronal (*A*) and axial (*B*) CT images show multiple odontogenic keratocysts present in the right and left maxillary premolar regions and the right mandibular molar-ramus region (*asterisks*). Note the calcification of the falx cerebri (*arrow*).

outer cortical plates. The presence of internal keratin may give the lesion a hazy appearance. Tooth displacement and root resorption are noted occasionally. Cortical perforation is a common feature.[9] The mandibular canal may be displaced inferiorly. In the maxilla, the lesion can expand into and occupy the entire maxillary sinus. Because of their keratin content, these lesions have a low-to-intermediate signal intensity on T1-weighted MR images and a heterogenous high signal intensity on T2-weighted images.[10]

Lateral Periodontal Cyst

Definition and clinical features
The lateral periodontal cyst is a developmental odontogenic cyst originating from remnants of the dental lamina in the periodontal ligament along the lateral root surface. The lesion is typically asymptomatic and is detected during a routine radiographic examination. It usually develops during the fifth through seventh decades of life. Most cases occur in the premolar-canine-lateral incisor area of jaws. The mandible is involved more commonly than the maxilla. The cyst tends to remain small, rarely exceeding 1 cm in diameter.

Imaging features
Radiographs reveal a round or ovoid well-defined interradicular radiolucency, often with a sclerotic margin (**Fig. 10**). Effacement of the adjacent lamina dura may occur. The buccal cortical plate may exhibit moderate expansion. There is a little tendency for the lesion to displace the adjacent teeth. The lesion may occasionally appear as a cluster of small cysts, in which case it is termed *botryoid odontogenic cyst*.

Glandular Odontogenic Cyst (Sialo-Odontogenic Cyst)

Definition and clinical features
Glandular odontogenic cyst is a rare type of developmental cyst that derives from odontogenic epithelium. Histologically, the lesion shows characteristic salivary gland features such as mucus-producing cells. It is most common in middle-aged adults, with a peak prevalence in the sixth decade of life. Men and women are affected equally. The lesion occurs more frequently in the mandible, with a strong predilection

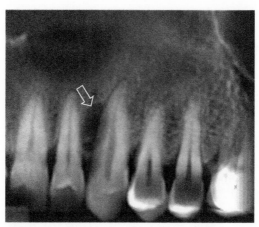

Fig. 10. Lateral periodontal cyst. Regional reformatted panoramic image from small field of view CBCT volume shows a well-defined, ovoid, radiolucent lesion over the midroot region of the lateral incisor and cuspid (*arrow*). CBCT, cone-beam computed tomography. (*Courtesy of* Marcel Noujeim, DDS, San Antonio, TX)

for the anterior region. This cyst often exhibits an aggressive behavior with a high recurrence rate.[11]

Imaging features
Radiographically, the lesion may present as a well-demarcated unilocular or multilocular radiolucency, with a smooth or scalloped border (**Fig. 11**). Lesions with a multilocular appearance may resemble an ameloblastoma. The lesion often expands and erodes the outer cortical bone and may displace the roots of teeth but it usually does not cause root resorption.[11]

Nasopalatine Duct Cyst (Incisive Canal Cyst)

The nasopalatine duct cyst is the most common nonodontogenic cyst of the jaws, representing approximately 12% of all cases of jaw cysts.[12] The lesion results from cystic degeneration of embryonic epithelial remnants in the nasopalatine canal. It is most common in the third to sixth decades of life, and the male-to-female ratio is almost 3:1. Presenting symptoms may include swelling, discharge, and pain.

Imaging features
The lesion presents as a well-circumscribed radiolucency between and apical to the maxillary central incisors. It usually has a round or ovoid shape with a thin rim of cortical bone (**Fig. 12**A–C). Some lesions may show a heart shape because of superimposition of the anterior nasal spine. This cyst frequently causes the roots of the central incisors to diverge. Root resorption is uncommon. The lesion may expand the outer cortical plates and elevate the nasal floor as it enlarges.

Nasolabial Cyst

Definition and clinical features
Nasolabial cyst (also referred to as nasoalveolar cyst) is a rare developmental cyst that occurs in the nasolabial fold deep to the ala of the nose. It is thought to originate from entrapped epithelium within the fusion lines of the nasal and maxillary processes or from embryonic remnants of the nasolacrimal duct. Nasolabial cysts may develop at any age but they are most commonly diagnosed in the fourth and fifth decades of

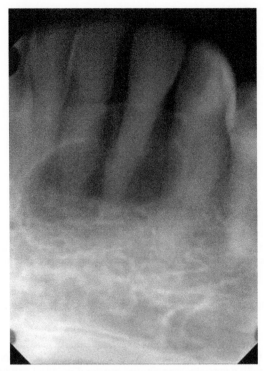

Fig. 11. Glandular odontogenic cyst in the anterior mandible. Periapical film shows a well-defined, multilocular radiolucent lesion with a smooth corticated margin.

life. Women are affected 3 times as often as men. Most lesions are unilateral, although bilateral cases have been reported.[13]

Imaging features
On imaging, a nasolabial cyst appears as a well-defined ovoid cystic mass in the soft tissues of the face deep to the lateral margin of the nose (**Fig. 13**A–D). The lesion may cause pressure erosion of the adjacent surface of maxilla.[14]

Ameloblastoma

Definition and clinical features
Ameloblastomas are benign, slowly growing, locally aggressive tumors of odontogenic epithelial origin. They are the second most common odontogenic tumors, following

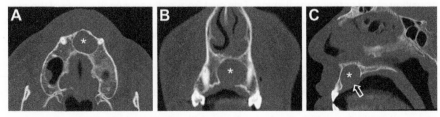

Fig. 12. Nasopalatine duct cyst. Axial (A), coronal (B), and sagittal (C) CT images of a naso-palatine duct cyst positioned palatal to maxillary incisors (asterisks). Note the erosion of the palatal cortex (arrow). (Courtesy of Matthew Parsons, MD, St. Louis, MO).

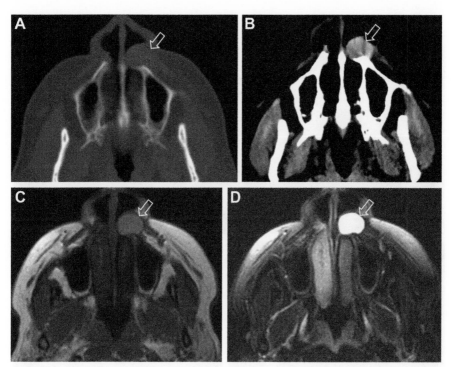

Fig. 13. Nasoalveolar cyst. Axial bone window (*A*) and soft tissue window (*B*) CT images show a well-defined soft-tissue mass deep to the left lateral nasal margin (*arrow*). The mass has caused erosion of the adjacent maxillary bone. Axial T1-weighted image (*C*) shows an intermediate signal intensity lesion (*arrow*), which is markedly hyperintense on axial T2-weighted image (*D*) (*arrow*). (*Courtesy of* Matthew Parsons, MD, St. Louis, MO).

odontomas. Ameloblastomas are divided into 3 types: solid/multicystic type (86%), unicystic type (13%), and extraosseous/peripheral type (1%).[15] The solid/multicystic variant occurs across a wide age range but it is discovered most frequently in patients aged between 20 and 40 years. There is no significant sex predilection. Approximately 80% of cases occur in the mandible, with a marked tendency to involve the posterior areas of the jaws. Small lesions are usually asymptomatic and are detected incidentally on routine radiographs. Large lesions may cause a painless swelling of the jaws. Ameloblastomas often tend to recur after surgical treatment.

Imaging features
The lesions may appear as unilocular or, more commonly, multilocular radiolucencies with curved, cortical borders. Multilocular lesions are often described as having either a "soap bubble" appearance (when the loculations are large and fewer in number) or a "honeycomb" appearance (when the loculations are small and numerous). The lesions sometimes are associated with an unerupted tooth. Most often there is rather marked expansion with thinning and erosion of the cortical plates. Tooth displacement and root resorption are common features (**Fig. 14**A–C). The computed tomography (CT) findings include hypodense cystic areas intermixed with hyperdense areas, reflecting the solid component of this lesion.[16] The unicystic ameloblastoma frequently appears as a pericoronal radiolucency, resembling a dentigerous cyst (**Fig. 15**A and B).

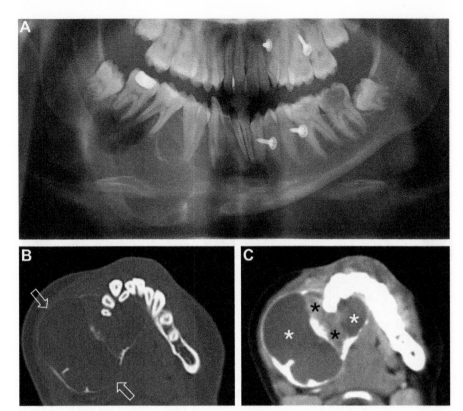

Fig. 14. Ameloblastoma of the mandible, solid/multicystic type. (*A*) Panoramic image shows a large, expansile, multilocular radiolucent lesion in the mandibular symphysis and body on the right side. Note the displacement and resorption of the adjacent teeth. (*B*) Axial CT (bone window setting) shows gross cyst-like expansion and thinning of the outer cortical plates leaving a thin shell of bone (*arrows*). (*C*) Axial contrast-enhanced CT (soft-tissue window setting) shows a complex cystic and solid tumor. The cystic portion is hypodense (*white asterisks*), whereas the solid portion is hyperdense (*black asterisks*).

Adenomatoid Odontogenic Tumor

Definition and clinical features

The adenomatoid odontogenic tumor accounts for 3% to 7% of all odontogenic tumors.[17] The origin of the tumor may be from enamel organ epithelium or from remnants of dental lamina. About two-thirds of all reported cases have been diagnosed during the second decade of life. The lesion occurs twice as frequently in the maxilla than the mandible, with a striking tendency to involve the anterior areas of the jaws. The male-to-female ratio is 1:2. The lesion is often asymptomatic, although large lesions may result in a painless swelling of the jaws. In approximately 75% of cases, the lesion is associated with an unerupted tooth, most often a canine.[15]

Imaging features

The radiographic appearance is that of a nonaggressive unilocular radiolucency with a well-defined cortical or sclerotic border. When associated with an impacted tooth, the lesion is attached to the tooth root at a point apical to the cementoenamel junction, a feature that may help distinguish it from a dentigerous cyst. Evidence of a radiopaque

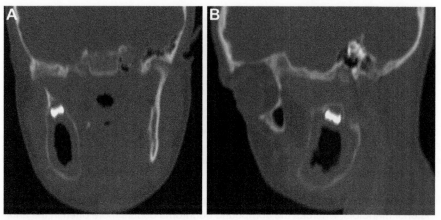

Fig. 15. Unicystic ameloblastoma. Coronal (*A*) and sagittal (*B*) CT scans show unilocular radiolucent lesion in the right ramus of the mandible. The lesion is causing expansion and thinning of the outer cortical plates as well as posterior-superior displacement of the mandibular third molar. A low density (*black area*) is seen within the lesion and represents an aspirated cystic lumen.

internal structure is found in about two-thirds of the cases (**Fig. 16**A and B). The radiopaque structure often has a flocculent appearance, resembling a snow-like pattern.[18] As the lesion enlarges, it may displace the adjacent teeth. The associated tooth may be displaced in an apical direction. There may be expansion with intact cortical plates. Root resorption is rarely noted.

Odontoma

Definition and clinical features
Odontomas are tumor-like malformations (hamartomas) consisting of variable amounts of dental tissues that are arranged in a disorganized fashion. Odontomas are subdivided into complex and compound types. Although both types may occur

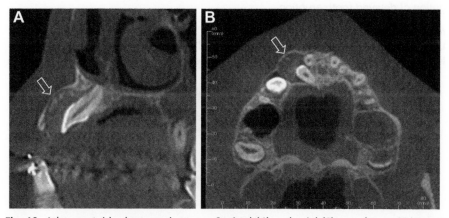

Fig. 16. Adenomatoid odontogenic tumor. Sagittal (*A*) and axial (*B*) cone-beam CT images show a unilocular, expansile lesion associated with the impacted lateral incisor (*arrows*). Note the clumped radiopaque flecks within the lesion.

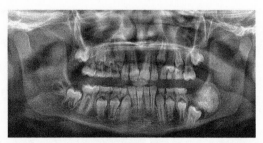

Fig. 17. Complex odontoma. Panoramic film shows a densely radiopaque mass overlying the crown of the mandibular left first molar, which has been displaced to the inferior border of the mandible. Note the thin radiolucent capsule and cortex at the periphery.

in any tooth-bearing area of the jaws, the complex odontoma is more often seen in the posterior mandible, whereas the compound odontoma occurs more often in the anterior maxilla. Compound odontoma is at least twice as common as complex odontoma. Most cases develop in children and adolescents. No sex predilection is noted. Odontomas are often incidental findings or they may result in delayed tooth eruption.

Imaging features
The complex odontoma is composed of an amorphous mass of tooth-like density and surrounded by a thin radiolucent capsule. The compound odontoma consists of a collection of miniature teeth (denticles), which is also surrounded by a soft tissue capsule. In both types, there is a cortical border immediately outside the radiolucent capsule (**Figs. 17** and **18**). Occasionally, lesions may show features of both complex and compound odontoma. Large odontomas can cause expansion of the jaw.

Ameloblastic Fibroma

Definition and clinical features
Ameloblastic fibromas are benign odontogenic tumors characterized by neoplastic proliferation of epithelial and mesenchymal tissues without the presence of dental hard tissues. The lesions usually originate in the first 2 decades of life without a significant sex predilection. Most cases develop in the premolar and molar area of the mandible. The lesion is usually asymptomatic and may be discovered during investigation of delayed tooth eruption.

Imaging features
Lesions appear as well-defined, often corticated, unilocular, or, less commonly, multilocular radiolucencies. Small lesions may appear as a unilocular outgrowth of the

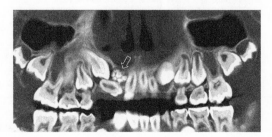

Fig. 18. Compound odontoma. Thin slice reformatted panoramic image from CBCT volume shows a compound odontoma (*arrow*) in the anterior maxilla interfering with eruption of the lateral incisor and cuspid. Note the numerous tooth-like structures and the radiolucent capsule.

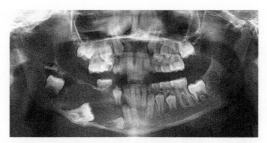

Fig. 19. Ameloblastic fibroma. Panoramic film of a well-defined radiolucent lesion involving the right mandibular body. The adjacent teeth are displaced in an apical direction.

follicle of an unerupted tooth. The tumor can expand bone but usually the outer cortex is maintained.[17] Because the tumor originates coronal to an unerupted tooth, it has a propensity to displace the associated tooth or teeth in an apical direction (**Fig. 19**).

Odontogenic Myxoma

Definition and clinical features

Odontogenic myxomas are uncommon intraosseous neoplasms, accounting for only 3% to 6% of odontogenic tumors. They most frequently occur in teenagers and young adults, and there is a slight female predilection.[19] About two-thirds of cases occur in the mandible, most often in the premolar and molar regions of the jaws. Large lesions cause a painless jaw expansion. The lesion is not encapsulated and appears to infiltrate the surrounding bone.

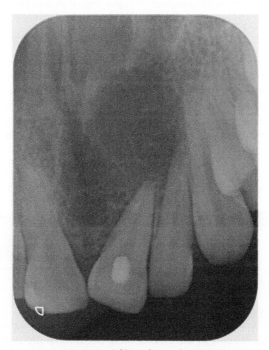

Fig. 20. Odontogenic myxoma. Periapical film of an odontogenic myxoma in the left anterior maxilla. Note the presence of a few thin straight septa. Moreover, note the displacement of the central and lateral incisors. (*Courtesy of* Nelson Silva, DDS, Concepción, Chile).

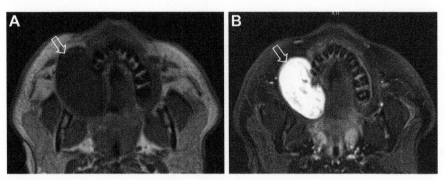

Fig. 21. Odontogenic myxoma of the maxilla. Axial T1-weighted (*A*) and T2-weighted (*B*) MR images show a large mass destroying the right posterior maxillary alveolus and expanding into the premaxillary soft tissues (*arrows*). The lesion has a low T1 signal intensity and high T2 signal intensity.

Imaging features

Odontogenic myxomas present as unilocular or multilocular radiolucent lesions. The periphery may be well defined with smooth or scalloped cortical border or may appear to be poorly defined. The bony septa forming the loculations usually are straight, thin, elongated, and lacy. These septa may produce a "tennis-racket" pattern (**Fig. 20**). Odontogenic myxomas occasionally expand bone and displace teeth but to a lesser degree than ameloblastomas.[18] Root resorption is rare. On MR imaging, odontogenic myxomas usually have a low-to-intermediate signal intensity on T1-weighted images and high signal intensity on T2-weighted images (**Fig. 21**A and B).[20]

Central Odontogenic Fibroma

Definition and clinical features

The central odontogenic fibroma is a rare intraosseous neoplasm of ectomesenchymal origin. The tumor demonstrates a wide age range, with a mean age of 40 years.[21] It is twice as common in women as in men. The mandible is involved more commonly than the maxilla. Although most mandibular lesions occur in the posterior region, maxillary lesions often are located anterior to the first molar. Smaller lesions are usually asymptomatic; larger lesions may be associated with painless swelling or mobility of teeth.

Imaging features

The tumor appears as a unilocular or multilocular radiolucency with well-defined borders. The internal septa may be granular and ill defined as those in central giant cell

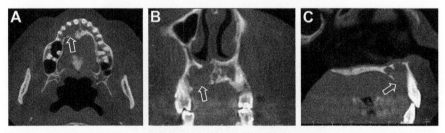

Fig. 22. Odontogenic fibroma of the maxilla. Axial (*A*), coronal (*B*), and sagittal (*C*) cone-beam CT images show a unilocular lesion (*arrows*) on the palatal aspect of the maxillary right incisors, cuspid, and first bicuspid. The lesion has destroyed the bone around the teeth without tooth displacement or resorption or significant expansion of the alveolar process.

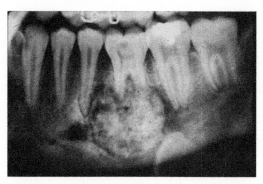

Fig. 23. Cementoblastoma. A cropped panoramic image shows a large radiopaque mass attached to the roots of the mandibular first molar and surrounded by a peripheral radiolucent band. There are mottled radiolucent areas within the mass. The roots of the first molar are partially resorbed.

granuloma, or may be fine and straight as those seen in odontogenic myxoma.[18] Sometimes, these lesions are associated with an impacted tooth. In rare instances, the lesion may contain radiopaque foci. Teeth may be either displaced or resorbed. The outer cortex may be expanded and thinned but remains intact. Some maxillary lesions have a characteristic behavior of extending in the periradicular area of the teeth without causing significant bone expansion (**Fig. 22**A–C).

Cementoblastoma

Definition and clinical features
Cementoblastoma is a rare, benign, odontogenic neoplasm of cementoblasts. The vast majority of cementoblastomas originate in the roots of the mandibular first molar and premolars. The neoplasm shows no gender preference and is encountered most frequently in children and young adults. Pain and swelling are the most common complaints. The involved tooth remains vital.[22]

Imaging features
Cementoblastoma typically appears as a well-circumscribed calcified mass that is attached to the tooth root and surrounded by a peripheral radiolucent band. The lesion may have a mottled appearance, with multiple radiolucent areas within the radiopaque mass (**Fig. 23**). A characteristic feature in some cases is the organization of the internal aspect into linear spicules of mineralized material radiating from the center in a spoke-wheel pattern.[23] The tumor usually causes root resorption of the involved tooth. If large, the lesion may cause expansion and perforation of the adjacent cortical plates. Inferior displacement of the mandibular canal may be seen.

SUMMARY

Benign odontogenic lesions frequently occur in the jaws and appear radiographically as well-defined unilocular or multilocular lucent areas, with a smooth or scalloped border. Most lesions are asymptomatic and first come to attention during a routine radiographic examination or because of painless swelling of the involved jaw. The radiologic analysis of these lesions may be approached by categorizing the lesion according to its anatomic location, periphery, internal aspect, and relationship to surrounding structures. Odontogenic lesions can be readily differentiated from nonodontogenic conditions because the epicenter of the former lesions is always located above the inferior alveolar canal in the mandible and below the sinus floor in the maxilla. These lesions are frequently associated with an impacted tooth, and the lesion's relationship to the tooth is an important differential diagnostic feature. Displacement and resorption of adjacent teeth is often seen. CT imaging is especially useful to reveal regions of perforation of the expanded cortical plates. In most cases, microscopic examination of the specimen is necessary to establish a definitive diagnosis.

DISCLOSURE

The authors declare that they have no conflict of interest.

REFERENCES

1. Jones AV, Craig GT, Franklin CD. Range and demographics of odontogenic cysts diagnosed in a UK population over a 30-year period. J Oral Pathol Med 2006; 35(8):500–7.
2. Shear M, Speight PM. Radicular cyst and residual cyst. In: Shear M, Speight PM, editors. Cysts of the oral and maxillofacial regions. 4th edition. Singapore, Singapore: Wiley Blackwell; 2007. p. 123–42.
3. White S, Pharoah M. Cysts. In: White S, Pharoah M, editors. Oral radiology: principles and interpretation. 7th edition. St Louis (MO): Elsevier; 2014. p. 334–57.
4. Bilodeau EA, Collins BM. Odontogenic cysts and neoplasms. Surg Pathol Clin 2017;10(1):177–222.
5. Scholl RJ, Kellett HM, Neumann DP, et al. Cysts and cystic lesions of the mandible: clinical and radiologic-histopathologic review. Radiographics 1999; 19:1107–24.
6. Lustmann J, Shear M. Radicular cysts arising from deciduous teeth. Review of the literature and report of 23 cases. Int J Oral Surg 1985;14(2):153–61.
7. El-Naggar AK, Chan JKC, Grandis JR, et al. World Health Organization classification of head and neck tumors. 4th edition. Lyon, France: IARC; 2017. p. 205–60.
8. Mortazavi H, Baharvand M. Jaw lesions associated with impacted tooth: A radiographic diagnostic guide. Imaging Sci Dent 2016;46(3):147–57.
9. Borghesi A, Nardi C, Giannitto C, et al. Odontogenic keratocyst: imaging features of a benign lesion with an aggressive behaviour. Insights Imaging 2018;9(5): 883–97.
10. Mosier KM. Lesions of the Jaw. Semin Ultrasound CT MR 2015;36(5):444–50.
11. Noffke C, Raubenheimer EJ. The glandular odontogenic cyst: clinical and radiological features; review of the literature and report of nine cases. Dentomaxillofac Radiol 2002;31(6):333–8.
12. Shear M, Speight PM. Nasopalatine duct (incisive canal) cyst. In: Shear M, Speight PM, editors. Cysts of the oral and maxillofacial regions. 4th edition. Singapore, Singapore: Wiley Blackwell; 2007. p. 108–18.
13. Lai WS, Lin YY, Chu YH, et al. Bilateral nasolabial cysts. Ear Nose Throat J 2019; 98(2):78.
14. Kaneda T, Weber AL, Scrivani SJ, et al. Cysts, tumors, and nontumorous lesions of the Jaw. In: Som PM, Curtin HD, editors. Head and neck imaging. 5th edition. St. Louis, MO: Mosby; 2011. p. 1469–546.
15. Neville BW, Damm DD, Allen CM, et al. Odontogenic cysts and tumors. In: Neville BW, Damm DD, Allen CM, et al, editors. Oral and maxillofacial pathology. 3rd edition. Philadelphia, PA: Saunders; 2008. p. 678–740.
16. Avril L, Lombardi T, Ailianou A, et al. Radiolucent lesions of the mandible: a pattern-based approach to diagnosis. Insights Imaging 2014;5(1):85–101.

17. Philipsen HP, Reichart PA, Nikai H. The adenomatoid odontogenic tumour (AOT): An update. Oral Med Pathol 1998;2:55–60.
18. White S, Pharoah M. Benign Tumors. In: White S, Pharoah M, editors. Oral radiology: principles and interpretation. 7th edition. St Louis (MO): Elsevier; 2014. p. 359–99.
19. Kaffe I, Naor H, Buchner A. Clinical and radiological features of odontogenic myxoma of the jaws. Dentomaxillofac Radiol 1997;26:299–303.
20. Kheir E, Stephen L, Nortje C, et al. The imaging characteristics of odontogenic myxoma and a comparison of three different imaging modalities. Oral Surg Oral Med Oral Pathol Oral Radiol 2013;116(4):492–502.
21. Allen CM, Hammond HL, Stimson PG. Central odontogenic fibroma, WHO type. A report of three cases with an unusual associated giant cell reaction. Oral Surg Oral Med Oral Pathol 1992;73:62–6.
22. Brannon RB, Fowler CB, Carpenter WM, et al. Cementoblastoma: an innocuous neoplasm? A clinicopathologic study of 44 cases and review of the literature with special emphasis on recurrence. Oral Surg Oral Med Oral Pathol Oral Radiol Endod 2002;93(3):311–20.
23. Langlais RP, Langland OE, Nortje CJ. Periapical radiopacities. In: Langlais RP, Langland OE, Nortje CJ, editors. Diagnostic imaging of the jaws. Baltimore: Williams and Wilkins; 1995. p. 529–64.

Imaging of Fibro-osseous Lesions and Other Bone Conditions of the Jaws

Noura Alsufyani, BDS, MSc, PhD, DipFHID[a,b,]*, Adel Alzahrani, BDS, MDS[a]

KEYWORDS

- Fibro-osseous • Fibrous dysplasia • Cemento-osseous dysplasia
- Ossifying fibroma • Central giant cell granuloma • Aneurysmal bone cyst
- Langerhans cell histiocytosis • Paget's disease

KEY POINTS

- Pathophysiology of fibro-osseous and other bone lesions affecting the jaws can be dysplastic, reactive, or neoplastic growths.
- The lesions discussed show common histology that can be insufficient for a diagnosis.
- Specific radiographic presentations can be depicted in advanced imaging and contribute to adequate diagnosis and management.

INTRODUCTION

The term "fibro-osseous lesions" is an umbrella term that is used to describe the histopathological picture of certain lesions where normal bone is replaced by fibrous tissue and immature bone or cementum-like structures. The term was employed as the histopathological features of these entities are indistinguishable.[1] However, as per the definition, several other inflammatory, reactive, benign, and malignant lesions would fit the description. In an effort to understand these entities, several classifications and reclassifications have been introduced in the World Health Organization (WHO), textbooks, and published articles.[2]

A key player to reaching the diagnosis is the oral and maxillofacial radiologist (OMFR). Despite attempts by OMFRs to publish work on classification and diagnosis, knowledge gap remains and is evidenced by continued confusion and published case reports with unwarranted management or intervention.[3,4]

---

[a] Department of Oral Medicine and Diagnostic Sciences, Oral & Maxillofacial Radiology, College of Dentistry, King Saud University, P.O. Box 60169, Riyadh 11545, Kingdom of Saudi Arabia; [b] Department of Medicine and Dentistry, School of Dentistry, University of Alberta, 5-522, Edmonton Clinic Health Academy, 11405 - 87 Avenue NW, T6G 1C9, Edmonton, AB, Canada
* Corresponding author. College of Dentistry, King Saud University, P.O. Box 60169, Riyadh 11545, Kingdom of Saudi Arabia.
E-mail address: alsufyan@ualberta.ca

Dent Clin N Am 68 (2024) 297–317
https://doi.org/10.1016/j.cden.2023.09.005
0011-8532/24/© 2023 Elsevier Inc. All rights reserved.

dental.theclinics.com

Consistency in nomenclature and understanding of disease mechanisms among the dental specialists are crucial to ensure proper diagnosis and management.

Fibro-osseous lesions and other bone lesions affecting the jaws are a group of diverse conditions that can be partially similar in clinical, radiographic, or histopathologic presentations. This review aims to discuss these lesions with focus on radiographic features to avoid diagnostic pitfalls.

CLASSIFICATION
Fibro-osseous Lesions

Fibrous dysplasia

Fibrous dysplasia (FD) is a benign skeletal disorder where normal bone tissue is substituted with fibrous tissue and disorganized woven bone. FD is somatic in nature and can be attributed to mutation of the GNAS1 gene.[5] FD can be monostotic (80%–85%) or polyostotic, typically below the age of 30.[6,7] The jaw bones, frontal, sphenoid, and zygoma are the principal bones involved in the skull and facial region and the maxilla is the most affected gnathic bone.

Polyostotic FD is linked with McCune-Albright syndrome, a condition that is almost exclusive to females.[8] McCune-Albright syndrome exhibits café au lait skin pigmentation, precocious puberty, hyperthyroidism, and excessive secretion of growth hormone. Mazabraud syndrome is a rarer syndrome characterized by the co-occurrence of polyostotic FD and intramuscular myxomas.[9]

FD in the craniofacial region is generally regarded as monostotic, even if multiple bones are affected, and is referred to as "craniofacial fibrous dysplasia." This is because FD is contiguous within the craniofacial bones affected and can cross the midline (**Fig. 1**A and B).[10] The incidence of monostotic craniofacial FD ranges from 10% to 25%, while craniofacial involvement in cases of polyostotic FD can reach rates as high as 90%.[11]

Most patients present with painless swelling and facial asymmetry; however, pain, pathologic fracture, and visual impairment have been reported.[7] Approximately 1% of

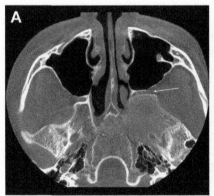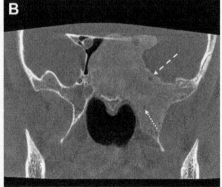

Fig. 1. Craniofacial FD. (*A*) Axial CBCT section and (*B*) coronal CBCT sections reveal FD in the body, pterygoid process, lesser and greater wings of the left sphenoid. Mild narrowing of the left pterygomaxillary fissure and pterygopalatine fossa (*arrow*) and vidian canal (*dotted arrow*). The distance between the left vidian canal and foramen rotundum (*dashed arrow*) is larger than on the left side. Note the enlargement but maintenance of the anatomic shape of the sphenoid bone and obliterated sphenoid sinus. CBCT, cone beam computed tomography; FD, fibrous dysplasia.

FD progresses into malignant sarcomatous transformation.[12] Significant risk factors for this transformation include exposure to radiation and the presence of McCune-Albright syndrome.[12]

Radiographically, FD typically demonstrates abnormal granular trabecular pattern classically described as "ground glass" (**Fig. 2**A–D). The borders are usually diffuse with a wide zone of transition between abnormal and normal bone; an important feature that is crucial in differentiating FD from cemento-ossifying fibroma (COF). Early lesions, however, can manifest with well-defined margins with mixed to low density.[13] Unlike benign neoplastic lesions, FD tends to cause bony expansion while maintaining the original anatomic shape of the involved bone. Loss of lamina dura and periodontal ligament space can be seen. Displacement of teeth and other adjacent structures (eg, sinonasal boundaries, orbital floor) can be observed.[14] The inferior alveolar canal may be displaced superiorly, in contrast to cystic lesions and benign tumors affecting the mandible (see **Fig. 2**A–D). This finding is considered by some authors as pathognomonic feature of FD.[15]

Concurrent presentation of simple bone cysts (SBCs) or aneurysmal bone cysts (ABCs) with fibro-osseous lesions has been reported.[16,17] Radiographic features of SBC of radiolucent spaces and scalloping can be seen within FD (**Fig. 3**A–C).

Cemento-osseous dysplasia

This is a non-neoplastic change affecting the tooth-bearing bone where normal bone is replaced by fibrous tissue and varying amounts of calcified material that increase as the lesion matures (**Fig. 4**A and B). Cemento-osseous dysplasia (COD) is common in

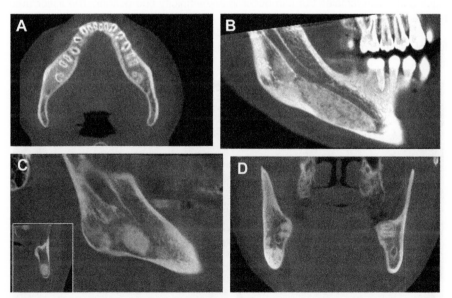

Fig. 2. Radiographic presentation of FD. CBCT images (*A*) Axial section, fine-granular bone pattern of FD in the right posterior mandibular molar area. (*B*) Corrected sagittal section reveals superior displacement of the mandibular canal. (*C*) Corrected sagittal section with inset coronal section, FD with cotton-wool density. (*D*) Coronal section, FD with a density similar to that of a dense bone island. Note the overall enlargement of the right mandibular body and ramus with maintenance of anatomic shape. FD, fibrous dysplasia; CBCT, cone beam computed tomography.

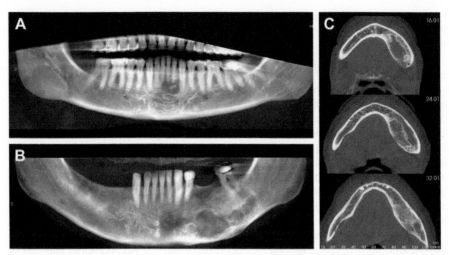

Fig. 3. Lesions existing with FD. Panoramic reconstruction from CBCT images (A) FD in the right mandibular angle and periapical cemento-osseous dysplasia (mixed stage) in the mandibular incisor region, (B) FD with simple bone cyst in the left mandibular body. (C) Axial CBCT images of the same case in (B) showing granular bone pattern and the large radiolucent component with expansion and thinning of the lingual cortex of mandible. FD, fibrous dysplasia; CBCT, cone beam computed tomography.

black and Asian females but can occur in any ethnicity and gender. The associated teeth are typically vital.

The term "cemento-" has been added and removed several times because the nature of calcified material cannot be confirmed to be cementum, only cementum-like.[1,2]

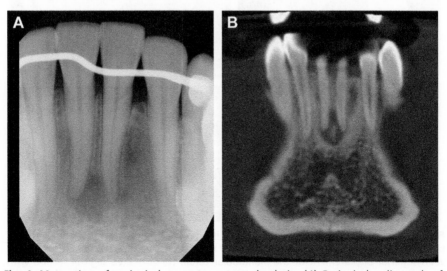

Fig. 4. Maturation of periapical cemento-osseous dysplasia. (A) Periapical radiograph of periapical radiolucency at mandibular incisors with intact PDL spaces. (B) Three years later, cementum-like calcifications are noted in the coronal CBCT section. CBCT, cone beam computed tomography; PDL, periodontal ligament.

There are 3 subjective presentations of this entity.

- Periapical COD: it affects the anterior teeth (can be bilateral).
- Focal COD: it affects the posterior teeth (can be bilateral).
- Florid COD: it shows extensive involvement of one or both jaws.

Radiographically, COD is usually well defined, with or without cortical outline, at the apical one-third of the root, and has internal calcifications similar to cortical bone or cementum.[18,19] As the lesion matures, a thin radiolucent rim, independent of the periodontal ligament space, is noted; however, it can be indiscernible in mature lesions (**Fig. 5A–D**). The cortical plates are usually unaffected but mild thinning, undulating endosteal surface, or nonconcentric expansion can be observed.[1,18]

Concomitant presentation of SBC with COD has been reported (12.7% prevalence).[16] The radiolucent background extends beyond the cementum-like calcifications and shows scalloping between the roots (**Fig. 6A and B**). Compared with solitary SBC, COD-associated SBC showed higher female predilection, presented in older age groups (fifth decade vs second), and were more likely to cause cortical expansion, root scalloping, and loss of lamina dura.[16] It is hypothesized that the empty cavity in bone forms due to the low or inadequate osteoblast numbers in the bones of middle-aged women or because of the changing biomechanical properties of adolescent bone during growth.[16]

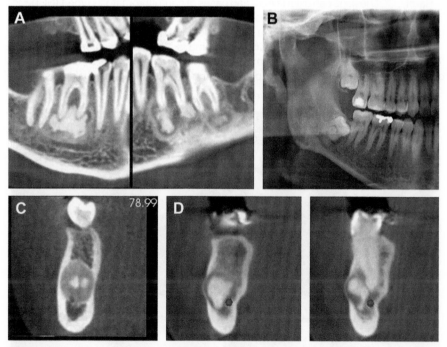

Fig. 5. Radiographic presentation of periapical/focal cemento-osseous dysplasia. (*A*) Corrected sagittal CBCT images showing bilateral, mixed lesions at the roots of mandibular molars. (*B*) Cropped panoramic radiograph showing similar lesion in an impacted third molar. CBCT bucco-lingual cross-sections of the right mandibular premolar area in (*C*) a combination of granular and cementum-like opacities and (*D*) irregular, nonconcentric cortical expansion, and no displacement of the mandibular canal. CBCT, cone beam computed tomography.

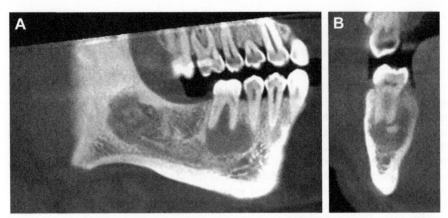

Fig. 6. Concomitant SBC with COD. CBCT images (*A*) corrected sagittal section, SBC scallop-ing between the roots of the right mandibular first molar, (*B*) cropped coronal section of the same lesion showing the cementum-like calcification. Note a second COD lesion in the third molar area. CBCT, cone beam computed tomography; COD, cemento-osseous dysplasia ; SBC, simple bone cyst.

Rarely, COD lesions can exist in ABC and cases of neurofibromatosis type 1 (NF1).[20,21] The cause is unknown, but theories favor altered local hemodynamics in ABC and gene alteration in NF1 affecting bone organization and reorganization (**Fig. 7**).[20,21]

A subcategory of COD that remains an enigma is "*familial gigantiform cementoma (FGC)*, aka familial florid COD or familial ossifying fibroma." This is a rare autosomal dominant condition with multiple, rapidly growing COD jaw lesions causing disfiguring

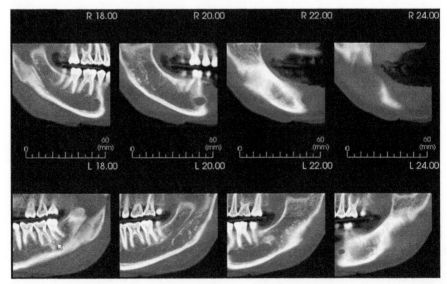

Fig. 7. COD with neurofibromatosis. Corrected sagittal CBCT images of bilateral wide mandibular canals and mental foramina. Note the mixed COD between the root apices of the left second and third molars (*arrow*). CBCT, cone beam computed tomography; COD, cemento-osseous dysplasia.

expansion in young subjects. Jaw lesions are excised to avoid excessive growth. Affected subjects may develop osteopenia and sustain long bone fractures. Diagnosing FGC is challenging because the COL1A2 mutation is not consistently found in FGC, sporadic gigantiform cementomas are reported (ie, lacking familial history), and its confusing heterogeneity with gnathodiaphyseal dysplasia, an autosomal dominant disorder in the ANO5 gene that features disfiguring fibro-osseous jaw lesions, long bone bowing with bone fragility, and recurrent fractures.[22–25]

Because of the abnormal bone metabolism, bone with COD is hypovascular and as such is prone to osteomyelitis (11% prevalence) if injury or infection is introduced by biopsy, dental disease, or treatment.[1,18,26] Alveolar ridge atrophy and presence of pulpal or periodontal disease increase the chances of secondary infection and the cementum-like calcifications would act as sequestra (**Fig. 8**A–C).[27] Maintaining good oral hygiene, arriving at proper diagnosis, and avoiding unnecessary intervention are key to avoid complications.

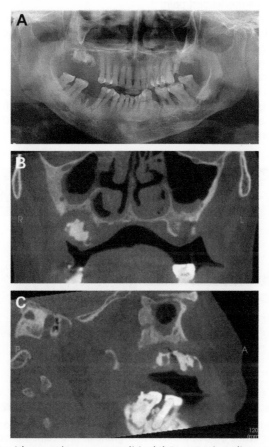

Fig. 8. Florid COD with secondary osteomyelitis. (*A*) Panoramic radiograph showing multifocal, mixed lesions periapical to the mandibular incisors and all molar teeth. CBCT images (*B*) Coronal section reveals "sequestrum" COD in the right posterior maxilla, resorption of alveolar crest, buccal and palatal plates of maxilla, sclerosis and thickening of the right maxillary sinus, (*C*) Sagittal section shows dense opacities periapical to the right mandibular molars. CBCT, cone beam computed tomography; COD, cemento-osseous dysplasia.

Cemento-ossifying/ossifying fibroma

COF is currently classified as a benign mesenchymal odontogenic tumor.[28] It is a thinly encapsulated benign neoplasm composed of dense fibrocellular tissue with irregular bony trabeculae or cementum-like material. The WHO previously grouped ossifying fibroma (OF) with COF but recently was reclassified as nonodontogenic origin under "benign fibro-osseous and chondro-osseous lesions."[29]

Juvenile OF is an uncommon variant presenting in middle childhood to adolescence and exhibits aggressive behavior with a higher likelihood of recurrence.[30] Multiple juvenile OFs can present in hyperparathyroidism-jaw tumor syndrome, which is an inherited disorder caused by a mutation in the tumor suppressor gene *CDC73*.[31]

Presence of multiple COF-like lesions warrants further investigations to rule out FGC, gnathodiaphyseal dysplasia, or hyperparathyroidism-jaw tumor syndrome.

COF is commonly observed in females during their third and fourth decades of life whereas males are slightly more affected by juvenile OF.[29,32] COF is mostly seen in the posterior mandible. The majority of cases are incidental or present as painless swelling and only 16% have experienced pain.[29]

Radiographically, COFs are well-defined, expansile lesions, with a thin border of radiolucent soft-tissue encapsulation. The lesions exhibit progressive calcification, initially manifesting as low-density areas that gradually become more radiopaque (**Fig. 9**A–C). Internally, the majority of lesions (58%) exhibit a ground-glass appearance, 26% of lesions were radiolucent, and 16% were sclerotic.[29]

COF may mimic FD radiographically. Unlike FD, which exhibits a tendency to merge with the adjacent bone, COF maintains well-defined boundaries with a distinct radiolucent band that separates it from the adjacent bone.[33] In addition, COF exhibits predominantly concentric expansion, which aligns with the anticipated pattern of benign

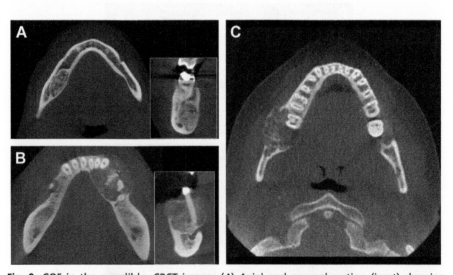

Fig. 9. COF in the mandible. CBCT images (A) Axial and coronal section (inset) showing mature COF with sclerotic border, a mixture of granular and cementum-like calcifications, and causing inferior displacement of the mandibular canal, (B) Axial and coronal section (inset) showing concentric expansion of COF with mesial displacement of the mandibular anterior teeth and narrowing of the mental foramen, (C) Axial section of COF presenting with scattered, wispy trabecular pattern. CBCT, cone beam computed tomography; COF, cemento-ossifying fibroma. (Images B and C are courtesy of Dr. Marcel Noujeim, DDS, MS, Oral and maxillofacial Radiologist, San Antonio, Texas, USA.).

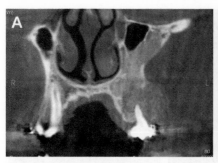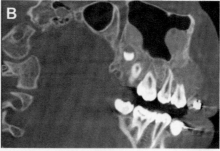

Fig. 10. COF of the maxilla. CBCT images A) Coronal section of COF in the left maxilla extending to the floor of maxillary sinus. Note the 2 bone patterns; fine-granular similar to "fibrous dysplasia" superiorly, fine-wispy and expansile at the alveolar process. B) Sagittal section showing concentric expansion affecting the buccal cortex of maxilla and anterior wall of maxillary sinus. Note apical root resorption of the maxillary left first premolar. CBCT, cone beam computed tomography; COF, cemento-ossifying fibroma. (Images are courtesy of Dr. Marcel Noujeim, DDS, MS, Oral and maxillofacial Radiologist, San Antonio, Texas, USA.).

neoplasms. Teeth displacement can occur as well as loss of lamina dura and root resorption. Maxillary lesions have the potential to cause significant displacement of the maxillary sinus, occasionally taking up nearly the entire volume of the sinus (**Fig. 10**A and B).

Giant Cell Lesions

Central giant cell granuloma

These lesions grow from bone cells with abundant giant cells and mostly affect the anterior mandible of patients younger than 30 years. There is a debate whether central giant cell granuloma (CGCG) is a benign neoplasm or reactive of unknown stimulus. However, due to its unpredictable and sometimes aggressive nature, classifying it as a benign neoplasm is preferable. Although efforts were done to identify mutations and immunohistochemical markers to differentiate CGCG of the jaws from giant cell tumor of bone, these are not conclusive due to small sample size and variability in data.[34,35]

Radiographically, CGCG is usually well defined, thinly corticated, unilocular or multilocular with fine-wispy septae (**Fig. 11**A–C). Dependent on aggressive behavior, teeth displacement and resorption, cortical thinning and expansion can vary (**Fig. 12**A–D). The presence of CGCG in adults warrants biochemical tests to assess hypercalcemia, hypophosphatasia, and increased PTH (parathyroid hormone) to rule-out brown tumor of hyperparathyroidism.

CGCG can exist with other lesions and become a hybrid CGCG. Common co-exiting lesions are central odontogenic fibroma (35.9%), central OF (28.2%), and FD (17.9%).[36] Radiographically, hybrid CGCG tends to blend with the coexisting lesion except for the radiopaque lesions of FD, melorheostosis, and Paget's disease of bone (PD), where CGCG features are clearly evident.[36]

Cherubism

Cherubism is an autosomal dominant condition due to mutations in the SH3BP2 gene where bilateral CGCG present in the posterior jaws. Although thought to be familial, hereditary and sporadic cases have been reported. It is a disease of childhood where CGCG causes significant bilateral expansion, giving rise to the facial appearance of

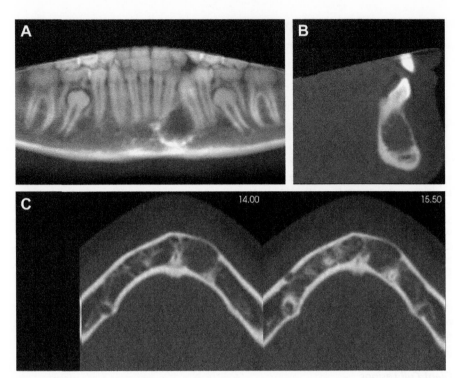

Fig. 11. CGCG. CBCT images (*A*) Cropped panoramic reconstruction of a 14-year-old female with CGCG in the left mandible causing displacement and delayed eruption of the left canine. (*B*) sagittal and (*C*) axial sections showing subtle wisps of fine-granular bone, undulating periphery, mild thinning, and expansion of the buccal cortex of mandible. CBCT, cone beam computed tomography; CGCG, central giant cell granuloma.

the chubby-cheeked little angels "cherubs." Jaw enlargement continues to puberty then tends to regress. Cherubism may be associated with neurofibromatosis type 1, fragile X syndrome, and Noonan-like syndrome.[37]

The radiographic appearance is characteristic; bilateral, well-defined, multilocular, and expansile radiolucent lesions. The epicenter of the lesions is in the posterior aspect of the jaws, resulting in anterior displacement of the teeth (**Fig. 13**A–C). The lesions can cause displacement of the maxillary sinuses and may extend to the condylar heads.[38]

Aneurysmal bone cyst

ABC is a benign, non-neoplastic, expansile, osteolytic lesion. It is composed of multiple blood-filled spaces separated by fibrous septa containing fibroblasts, reactive woven bone, and osteoclast-like giant cells.[39] ABCs can arise de novo or in pre-existing lesions such as FD, COD, CGCG, chondrosarcoma, or osteosarcoma.[21]

Most ABCs occur in children and young adults, with no significant gender predilection. Lesions are most common in the posterior mandible. They usually present as a relatively rapidly growing, painful jaw mass.

Radiographically, the lesion presents as a multilocular, or less commonly, unilocular radiolucency associated with marked expansion ("ballooning") and thinning of the outer cortical plates. The margins may be well defined or ill defined. Lesions often

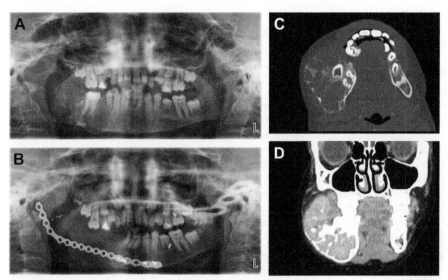

Fig. 12. Aggressive central giant cell granuloma of the mandible. Panoramic radiographs (*A*) of a 10-year-old boy showing multilocular, expansile radiolucency causing teeth displacement, (*B*) Four months postoperative jaw resection. Multidetector computed tomography (*C*) Axial bone window and (*D*) coronal soft tissue window showing a large, expansile, multilocular, low-attenuation lesion with multiple thin septae emanating from periphery to center. Note granular bone matrix surrounding the teeth.

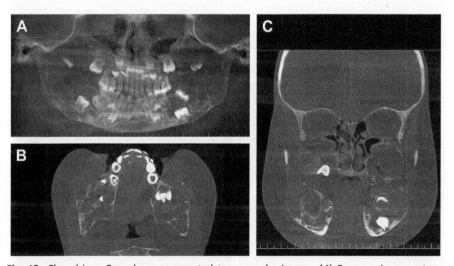

Fig. 13. Cherubism. Cone beam computed tomography images (*A*) Panoramic reconstruction showing bilateral, multilocular, expansile radiolucencies in the posterior maxilla and mandible. The condylar heads are spared. Note the anterior displacement of the unerupted molars bilaterally. (*B*) Axial section showing mandibular lesions with fine septae, some emanating at 90° toward the center of the lesion. (*C*) Coronal image showing the expansile lesions with extra-oral swelling of cheeks and involvement of the maxillary sinuses. (Images are courtesy of Dr. Marcel Noujeim, DDS, MS, Oral and maxillofacial Radiologist, San Antonio, Texas, USA.).

have wispy, ill-defined septa similar to those of a CGCG. Tooth displacement and root resorption may occur.[40] On MRI, typically there are multiple cystic components and fluid-fluid levels (**Fig. 14**A–D).

Other Osseous Conditions

Paget's disease

PD, also referred to as osteitis deformans, is a chronic disorder characterized by abnormal bone remodeling due to dysregulated osteoclast and osteoblast activity, causing structurally defective bone and marrow fibrosis. PD undergoes 3 temporal phases: lytic, mixed lytic-blastic, and blastic. Although the disease can affect various bones, the involvement of the jaws is relatively rare compared to that of the skull, pelvis, or femur.

PD typically affects people between the ages 55 and 75, with a rare incidence among those under the age of 40. Higher prevalence of PD is found in individuals of Anglo-Saxon descent residing in Europe, North America, Australia, and New Zealand,

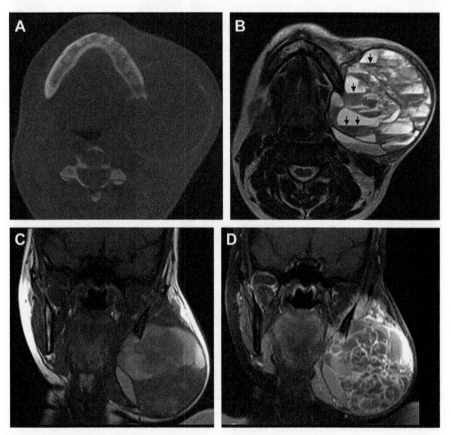

Fig. 14. ABC. (*A*) Axial CBCT image shows expansile, low-density lesion with undulating borders in the left posterior mandible. (*B*) Axial T2-weighted MRI showing hyperintense multicystic appearance with fluid-fluid levels (*arrowheads*) in the ABC. Coronal pregadolinium (*C*) and postgadolinium (*D*) T1-weighted MRI of the ABC showing contrast enhancement. ABC, aneurysmal bone cyst; CBCT, cone beam computed tomography (Reproduced with permission from Elsevier)[40]

while it is notably rare in Asia, Africa, and Scandinavia. Males are slightly more susceptible than females.[41]

Bone pain is a common symptom at diagnosis and blood test reveals elevated alkaline phosphatase levels. Potential complications include deformity and rare sarcomatous degeneration (<0.5%).[42] However, the 5-year survival rate for osteosarcoma arising from PD in the jaw is 21%, significantly lower than primary osteosarcoma of the jaw.[43]

Early lesions may manifest as radiolucencies that progress to a "ground-glass" or "cotton-wool" attenuation pattern and then mature to a uniformly sclerotic appearance with increased bone size. PD jaw lesions often show cortical and trabecular thickening, sclerotic alterations in alveolar bone, hypercementosis, and loss of lamina dura (**Fig. 15A–C**). Extragnathic features of PD include well-defined lytic cranial lesions, referred to as osteoporosis circumscripta, as well as the "tam-o'-shanter"

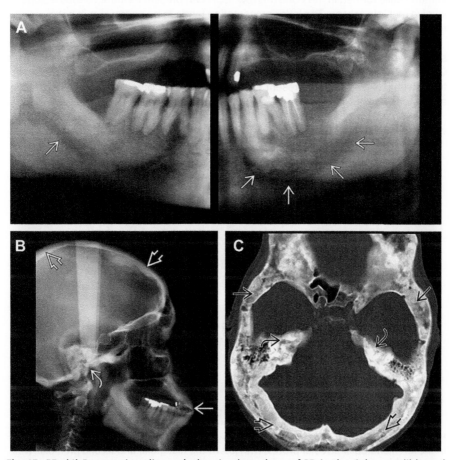

Fig. 15. PD. (*A*) Panoramic radiograph showing late phase of PD in the right mandible and early phase in the left mandible noted by the radiolucent area. Note hypercementosis in the right mandibular molars. (*B*) Lateral skull radiograph showing thickening of the diploic space, sclerosis of skull base, and flaring of the anterior teeth. (*C*) Axial bone MDCT showing mixed phase of PD in calvarium and cranial base with cotton-wool pattern in the squamous temporal and occipital bones. MDCT, multidetector computed tomography; PD, Paget's disease. (Reproduced with permission from Elsevier.)[45]

sign due to expansion of the diploic space and platybasia caused by the skull base softening. Bone scintigraphy can aid in diagnosing PD by revealing widespread radio-tracer uptake in the mandible, creating a "black beard" appearance known as the "Lincoln sign."[13]

Lesions involving the alveolar process can mimic florid COD; however, a distinguishing characteristic is their extension into the basal bone. PD imaging features can resemble FD; however, age of onset (young in FD), bilateral presentation (FD usually is unilateral), and PD changes in the skull can aid differentiation.

Langerhans cell histiocytosis

Formerly known as histiocytosis X, Langerhans cell histiocytosis (LCH) includes Letterer-Siwe disease, Hand-Schuller-Christian disease, and eosinophilic granuloma. This rare spectrum is characterized by the proliferation of Langerhans cells, dendritic immune cells formed in the bone marrow. LCH can present as intraosseous lesions or involve multiple organs. The latter presentation tends to be aggressive in behavior and requires radiation or chemotherapy.[44]

The average age of LCH is 14 years (range: 11 months–59 years) and although some studies report male predilection, others show the opposite.[44] LCH of the bone targets vertebrae, long bones, the mandible in children, the cranium and ribs in adults. Patients with jaw lesions may present with pain, tooth mobility, gingival bleeding, ulcerations, or swelling.

Most gnathic lesions present in the mandible as "scooped-out" bony destruction, with periosteal reaction parallel to the original cortex. There may be peripheral bone

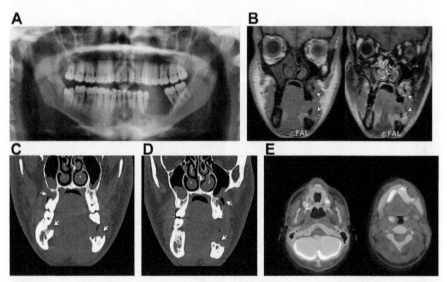

Fig. 16. LCH. (A) Panoramic radiograph of a 23-year-old male shows large radiolucent defect in the left mandibular alveolar process with loss of the first molar and second premolar. Note the saucer shape of the bone destruction. A similar but smaller lesion is noted on the contralateral side. Bilateral, ill-defined radiolucencies are noted in the maxillary premolar-molar area. Coronal MR images (B) T1WI and T1+C show isointense signal similar to muscle with mild enhancement (arrowheads). Coronal MDCT bone-windows (C) and (D) showing multifocal "punched-out" osteolytic lesions in the maxilla and mandible (arrows). (E) Nuclear medicine images (PET-FDG) reveal high uptake in the LCH lesions. FDG, fluorodeoxyglucose; LCH, Langerhan's cell histiocytosis; MDCT, multidetector computed tomography.

Table 1
Summary of common radiographic features of fibro-osseous and other bone lesions affecting the jaws

	Location	Periphery	Internal Structure	Effects on Surrounding Structures	Key Points
FD	Monostotic: Maxilla>mandible Unilateral Polyostotic: Multiple bones Craniofacial: Multiple cranial bones	Ill-defined, blending Early lesions are well defined	Granular (ground-glass) appearance Can be mixed with sclerotic areas and cystic cavities	Nonconcentric expansion (maintain the overall shape) +/– displacement of teeth, sinonasal structures, orbit, IANC Loss of lamina dura and thin PDL space	Polyostotic FD is associated with McCune-Albright syndrome Superior displacement of the IANC is pathognomonic
COD (Periapical, focal, and florid)	Mandible>maxilla Unilateral or bilateral Solitary or multiple Florid type: extensive involvement of one or both jaws	Well defined +/– cortical boundary	3 stages: RL, mixed, RO Radiopacities similar to cortical bone or cementum Calcified material can have swirling or fine-granular pattern	Minimal, nonconcentric cortical expansion Normal PDL space	Generally maintains radiolucent rim Can coexist with simple bone cyst Risk of secondary osteomyelitis Epicenter above IANC
COF	Mandible>maxilla	Well defined with thin radiolucent rim	Variable degree of RO depending on lesion maturity Can be granular, resembling fibrous dysplasia	Concentric expansion Displacement of teeth, maxillary sinus, IANC Root resorption	Juvenile subtypes exhibit aggressive behavior Well-defined margin helps to differentiate COF from FD Multiple lesions → consider hyperparathyroidism-jaw tumor syndrome
Central giant cell granuloma	Mandible>maxilla Unilateral or bilateral (brown tumors)	Well defined +/– thin cortical boundary	Unilocular or multilocular RL (fine septae, ± emanate from peripheral boundary to center at right angle)	Variable cortical expansion +/– teeth displacement or resorption	Can present with radiopacities when hybrid with bone dysplasia

(continued on next page)

Table 1
(continued)

	Location	Periphery	Internal Structure	Effects on Surrounding Structures	Key Points
Cherubism	Mandible>maxilla Bilateral Epicenter: posterior	Well defined +/− thin cortical boundary	Unilocular RL (rare) Multilocular RL: multiple, fine-granular septae, overall sclerotic or "fibro-osseous matrix" appearance	Expansile Anterior displacement of teeth	Regress in adulthood
Aneurysmal bone cyst	Mandible>maxilla Solitary	Well defined +/− cortical boundary	Multilocular RL (fine septae) Vascular, solid, and mixed types	Very expansile Teeth displacement or resorption	Can coexist with bone dysplasia and other benign tumors Angiography needed to verify feeding vessels
Paget's disease	Multiple bones Rare in the jaws Maxilla>mandible Bilateral	The entire bone is affected	3 stages: RL, mixed, RO RO: cotton-wool or sclerotic	Bone enlargement Teeth displacement and hypercementosis	Look for lytic lesions in the skull and increased diploic space Increased serum alkaline phosphatase
Langerhans cell histiocytosis	Solitary or multifocal Alveolar, intraosseous, or multiorgan Can affect tooth follicle	Well defined Noncorticated Scooped-out or lobulated	RL Variable fluid content and enhancement	Cortical expansion +/− sclerosis of surrounding bone +/− periosteal reaction parallel to cortical plate +/− displace tooth germ	Look for other lesions in bone or organs Wide range of presentation based on behavior; aggressive benign to indolent malignant

Abbreviations: COD, cemento-osseous dysplasia; COF, cemento-ossifying fibroma; FD, fibrous dysplasia; IANC, inferior alveolar nerve canal; RL, radiolucent; RO, radiopaque; PDL, periodontal ligament.

Table 2
Diagnostic tree of fibro-osseous and other bone lesions affecting the jaws based on common radiographic appearance

Classification	Entities	Ddx
RL Solitary — Unilocular — Expansile — Concentric	COF, CGCG, ABC, LCH	Ameloblastoma, OKC, residual cyst, fibrous scar. Malignancy (destructive)
RL Solitary — Unilocular — Nonexpansile — Nonconcentric	Early PCD, SBC	—
RL Solitary — Unilocular — Nonexpansile	Early PCD, SBC, LCH	Small odontogenic cyst or tumor. Periodontal disease (crestal). Malignancy (destructive)
RL Solitary — Multilocular	CGCG and ABC	Ameloblastoma, odontogenic myxoma, OKC (less expansile). Periodontal disease (crestal). Malignancy (destructive)
RL Multifocal — Unilocular	COD, CGCG (brown tumor), LCH	Periapical granuloma/cyst. Periodontal disease. Malignancy (destructive)
RL Multifocal — Multilocular	Cherubism	—
Mixed or Predominately RO — Well defined — Expansile — Concentric	COF, hybrid CGCG	Cementoblastoma (periapical), CEOT, ameloblastic fibro-odontoma, complex odontoma, COC, AOT
Mixed or Predominately RO — Well defined — Expansile — Nonconcentric	COD	Healed SBC, odontoma (tooth-like density)
Mixed or Predominately RO — Well defined — Nonexpansile	COD	Healed SBC, odontoma (tooth-like density)
Mixed or Predominately RO — Diffuse	Monostotic FD	Osteomyelitis (sequestra + parallel periosteal bone reaction), Osteogenic sarcoma (destructive, sun-ray periosteal bone reaction)
Mixed or Predominately RO — Multifocal — Above IANC	Florid COD	—
Mixed or Predominately RO — Multifocal — Beyond IANC	Paget's, Polyostotic FD, FGC, HPT-JT	Gardner's syndrome, Osteopetrosis

Abbreviations: ABC, aneurysmal bone cyst; AOT, adenomatoid odontogenic tumor; CEOT, calcifying epithelial odontogenic tumor; CGCG, central giant cell granuloma; COC, calcifying odontogenic cyst; COD, cemento-osseous dysplasia; COF, cemento-ossifying fibroma; Ddx, differential diagnosis; FD, fibrous dysplasia; FGC, familial gigantic cementoma; HPT-JT, hyperparathyroidism jaw tumors; IANC, inferior alveolar nerve canal; LCH, Langerhans cell histiocytosis; OKC, odontogenic keratocyst; PCD, periapical osseous dysplasia; RL, radiolucent; RO, radiopaque; SBC, simple bone cyst.

sclerosis (**Fig. 16**A–E). The bone destruction from alveolar LCH lesions may appear very similar to periodontal disease. Solitary intraosseous lesions can mimic squamous cell carcinoma and metastatic disease. Definitive diagnosis of bone LCH is confirmed by histopathological and immunohistochemical examinations.

RADIOGRAPHIC APPEARANCE AND DIFFERENTIAL DIAGNOSES

Fibro-osseous and other bone lesions affecting the jaws discussed in this review can have a wide range of radiographic features. Common features and important points are summarized in **Table 1**.

The radiographic differential diagnoses of fibro-osseous and other bone lesions affecting the jaws largely depend on periphery, distribution, internal structure, and effects on surrounding structures. It is important to take into consideration the clinical presentation and chronologic development of the lesion. As such, entities to be considered in the differential diagnosis can be anywhere from reactive to malignant diseases. Diagnostic tree of the lesions is provided in **Table 2**.

SUMMARY

Fibro-osseous and other bone lesions affecting the jaws discussed in this review can have overlapping histopathological picture or radiographic features. The clinical-radiographic correlation is key to understand the biological behavior and follow a diagnostic tree that culminates to proper management. Diversity in clinical-radiographic-histopathologic presentation along with hybrid occurrences of such lesions remains a challenge. The contribution of OMFRs in the comprehensive clinical and radiographic assessment is crucial to arriving at a diagnosis, recommending biopsy sites that can be representative of the lesion, and suggesting watchful waiting in cases where an intervention would be detrimental to the patient.

CLINICS CARE POINTS

- Analysis of all the correlating clinical, radiographic, and histological factors in a case is key. The ultimate goal is to provide the patient with accurate diagnosis and facilitate adequate management.
- Histopathologic examination is not needed or may even be contraindicated in some bone conditions (e.g., COD).
- Hybrid presentations may complicate the diagnostic process. Thorough selection of imaging modalities prior to biopsy elucidates the different tissues and lesion behavior.
- The oral and maxillofacial radiologist can explain the lesion's growth pattern, internal structure, and extent using different imaging modalities that reveal different aspects of the lesion.

DISCLOSURE

The authors have nothing to disclose.

REFERENCES

1. Nelson BL, Phillips BJ. Benign Fibro-Osseous Lesions of the Head and Neck. Head Neck Pathol 2019;13(3):466–75.

2. El-Naggar AK, Chan JKC, Takata T, et al. The fourth edition of the head and neck World Health Organization blue book: editors' perspectives. Hum Pathol 2017; 66:10–2.

3. Brody A, Zalatnai A, Csomo K, et al. Difficulties in the diagnosis of periapical translucencies and in the classification of cemento-osseous dysplasia. BMC Oral Health 2019;19(1):139.

4. Decolibus K, Shahrabi-Farahani S, Brar A, et al. Cemento-Osseous Dysplasia of the Jaw: Demographic and Clinical Analysis of 191 New Cases. Dent J 2023;11(5).

5. Cohen MM. Fibrous dysplasia is a neoplasm. Am J Med Genet 2001;98(4):290–3.

6. Andreu-Arasa VC, Chapman MN, Kuno H, et al. Craniofacial Manifestations of Systemic Disorders: CT and MR Imaging Findings and Imaging Approach. Radiographics 2018;38(3):890–911.

7. MacDonald-Jankowski D. Fibrous dysplasia: A systematic review. Dentomaxillofacial Radiol 2009;38(4):196–215.

8. Feller L, Wood NH, Khammissa RA, et al. The nature of fibrous dysplasia. Head Face Med 2009;5(1). https://doi.org/10.1186/1746-160X-5-22.

9. Majoor BCJ, Van De Sande MAJ, Appelman-Dijkstra NM, et al. Prevalence and clinical features of mazabraud syndrome: A multicenter european study. Journal of Bone and Joint Surgery - American 2019;101(2):160–8.

10. Rahman AMA, Madge SN, Billing K, et al. Craniofacial fibrous dysplasia: Clinical characteristics and long-term outcomes. Eye 2009;23(12):2175–81.

11. Ricalde P, Magliocca KR, Lee JS. Craniofacial Fibrous Dysplasia. Oral Maxillofac Surg Clin North Am 2012;24(3):427–41.

12. Stanton RP. Surgery for fibrous dysplasia. J Bone Miner Res 2007;22(SUPPL. 2). https://doi.org/10.1359/JBMR.06S220.

13. Holmes KR, Holmes RD, Martin M, et al. Practical Approach to Radiopaque Jaw Lesions. Radiographics 2021;41(4):E1164–85.

14. MacDonald-Jankowski D, Yeung R, Li T, et al. Computed tomography of fibrous dysplasia. Dentomaxillofacial Radiol 2004;33(2):114–8.

15. Petrikowski CG, Pharoah MJ, Lee L, et al. Radiographic differentiation of osteogenic sarcoma, osteomyelitis, and fibrous dysplasia of the jaws. Oral Surgery, Oral Medicine, Oral Pathology, Oral Radiology, and Endodontology. 1995;80(6): 744–50.

16. Chadwick JW, Alsufyani NA, Lam EWN. Clinical and radiographic features of solitary and cemento-osseous dysplasia-associated simple bone cysts. Dentomaxillofac Radiol 2011;40(4):230–5.

17. Koketsu Y, Tanei T, Kuwabara K, et al. Secondary aneurysmal bone cyst of the frontal bone with fibrous dysplasia showing rapid expansion: a case report. Nagoya J Med Sci 2023;85(2):395–401.

18. Alsufyani NA, Lam EWN. Osseous (Cemento-osseous) Dysplasia of the Jaws: Clinical and Radiographic Analysis. J Can Dent Assoc 2011;77.

19. Ahmad M, Gaalaas L. Fibro-Osseous and Other Lesions of Bone in the Jaws. Radiol Clin North Am 2018;56(1):91–104.

20. Friedrich RE, Reul A. Periapical Cemento-osseous Dysplasia Is Rarely Diagnosed on Orthopantomograms of Patients with Neurofibromatosis Type 1 and Is Not a Gender-specific Feature of the Disease. Anticancer Res 2018;38(4):2277–84.

21. Yeom HG, Yoon JH. Concomitant cemento-osseous dysplasia and aneurysmal bone cyst of the mandible: a rare case report with literature review. BMC Oral Health 2020;20(1):276.

22. Moshref M, Khojasteh A, Kazemi B, et al. Autosomal dominant gigantiform cementoma associated with bone fractures. Am J Med Genet 2008;146A(5):644–8.

23. Prasad C, Kumar KA, Balaji J, et al. A family of familial gigantiform cementoma: clinical study. J Maxillofac Oral Surg 2022;21(1):44–50.
24. Nel C, Yakoob Z, Schouwstra CM, et al. Familial florid cemento-osseous dysplasia: a report of three cases and review of the literature. Dentomaxillofacial Radiol 2021;50(1).
25. MacDonald DS. Classification and nomenclature of fibro-osseous lesions. Oral Surg Oral Med Oral Pathol Oral Radiol 2021;131(4):385–9.
26. Alsufyani N, Lam E. Cemento-osseous dysplasia of the jaw bones: key radiographic features. Dentomaxillofacial Radiol 2011;40(3):141–6.
27. Nadler C, Perschbacher SE, Septon D, et al. Important radiographic features in the identification of osseous dysplasia–related osteomyelitis. Oral Surg Oral Med Oral Pathol Oral Radiol 2021;131(6):730–7.
28. Speight PM, Takata T. New tumour entities in the 4th edition of the World Health Organization Classification of Head and Neck tumours: odontogenic and maxillofacial bone tumours. Virchows Arch 2018;472(3):331–9.
29. MacDonald-Jankowski D. Ossifying fibroma: a systematic review. Dentomaxillofacial Radiol 2009;38(8):495–513.
30. El-Mofty SK. Fibro-Osseous Lesions of the Craniofacial Skeleton: An Update. Head Neck Pathol 2014;8(4):432–44.
31. Torresan F, Iacobone M. Clinical Features, Treatment, and Surveillance of Hyperparathyroidism-Jaw Tumor Syndrome: An Up-to-Date and Review of the Literature. Int J Endocrinol 2019;2019:1–8.
32. El-Mofty S. Psammomatoid and trabecular juvenile ossifying fibroma of the craniofacial skeleton: Two distinct clinicopathologic entities. Oral Surgery, Oral Medicine, Oral Pathology, Oral Radiology, and Endodontology 2002;93(3):296–304.
33. Ahmad M, Gaalaas L. Fibro-Osseous and Other Lesions of Bone in the Jaws. Radiol Clin North Am 2018;56(1):91–104.
34. Gomes CC, Diniz MG, Bastos VC, et al. Making sense of giant cell lesions of the jaws (GCLJ): lessons learned from next-generation sequencing. J Pathol 2020;250(2):126–33.
35. Nagar SR, Bansal S, Jashnani K, et al. A Comparative Analysis of p63 Expression in Giant Cell Tumour (GCT), Central Giant Cell Granuloma (CGCG) and Peripheral Giant Cell Granuloma (PGCG). Head Neck Pathol 2020;14(3):733–41.
36. Alsufyani NA, Aldosary RM, Alrasheed RS, et al. A systematic review of the clinical and radiographic features of hybrid central giant cell granuloma lesions of the jaws. Acta Odontol Scand 2021;79(2).
37. Papadaki ME, Lietman SA, Levine MA, et al. Cherubism: best clinical practice. Orphanet J Rare Dis 2012;7(Suppl 1).
38. Beaman FD, Bancroft LW, Peterson JJ, et al. Imaging Characteristics of Cherubism. Am J Roentgenol 2004;182(4):1051–4.
39. Liu Y, Zhou J, Shi J. Clinicopathology and Recurrence Analysis of 44 Jaw Aneurysmal Bone Cyst Cases: A Literature Review. Front Surg 2021;8:678696.
40. Omami G, Mathew R, Gianoli D, et al. Enormous aneurysmal bone cyst of the mandible: case report and radiologic-pathologic correlation. Oral Surg Oral Med Oral Pathol Oral Radiol 2012;114(1):e75–9.
41. Charles JF, Siris ES, Roodman GD. Paget Disease of Bone. In: Primer on the metabolic bone diseases and disorders of Mineral metabolism. Wiley; 2018. p. 713–20. https://doi.org/10.1002/9781119266594.ch92.
42. Ralston SH. Paget's Disease of Bone. N Engl J Med 2013;368(7):644–50.
43. Cheng YSL, Wright JM, Walstad WR, et al. Osteosarcoma arising in Paget's disease of the mandible. Oral Oncol 2002;38(8):785–92.

44. Reisi N, Raeissi P, Harati Khalilabad T, et al. Unusual sites of bone involvement in Langerhans cell histiocytosis: a systematic review of the literature. Orphanet J Rare Dis 2021;16(1):1.

45. Petrikowski CG. Paget Disease. In: Koenig LJ, Tamimi D, Petrikowski CG, et al, editors. Diagnostic imaging: oral and maxillofacial. 2nd Edition. Elsevier; 2017. p. 449. https://doi.org/10.1016/B978-0-323-47782-6.50130-7.

Malignant Lesions of the Oral Region

Galal Omami, BDS, MSc, MDentSc, FRCD(C), Dip. ABOMR[a],*,
Melvyn Yeoh, MD, DMD[b]

KEYWORDS

- Mouth neoplasms • Mandible • Computed tomography • MRI

KEY POINTS

- Primary and metastatic malignancies may affect the jaws and mimic periapical inflammatory disease.
- Advanced imaging modalities play an important role in the preoperative evaluation and staging of oral region cancers.
- Computed tomography (CT) and MRI are invaluable in demonstrating the location and extent of the tumor, which is important in planning the surgical approach.
- PET-CT imaging is highly effective in detection of metastasis and recurrent disease.

INTRODUCTION

This article deals with diagnostic imaging of malignant neoplasms of the oral region. Most of these malignancies are squamous cell carcinomas (SCCs).[1] Other malignant lesions encountered in this region include sarcomas (eg, osteosarcoma, chondrosarcoma, rhabdomyosarcoma), salivary gland tumors (eg, mucoepidermoid carcinoma, adenoid cystic carcinoma, adenocarcinoma), malignancies of the hematopoietic system (eg, lymphoma, multiple myeloma), and metastases (**Box 1**).

Radiographic features that are suggestive of a malignant lesion include the following: ill-defined "moth-eaten" or permeative pattern of bone destruction, irregular widening of periodontal ligament space with destruction of the adjacent lamina dura, destructive soft-tissue mass, destruction of the supporting alveolar bone resulting in teeth "floating in space," periosteal bone formation, patchy bone sclerosis, enlargement of the dental follicle with destruction of the follicular cortex and displacement of the developing tooth crypts, "spiking" resorption of the tooth resulting in tapered narrowing of the root apex, enlargement of a recent extraction socket, and irregular

[a] Division of Oral Diagnosis, Oral Medicine, and Oral Radiology, Department of Oral Health Practice, University of Kentucky College of Dentistry, 770 Rose Street, MN320, Lexington, KY 40536, USA; [b] Division of Oral and Maxillofacial Surgery, University of Kentucky College of Dentistry, 770 Rose Street, D-528, Lexington, KY 40536, USA
* Corresponding author.
E-mail address: galal.omami@uky.edu

Dent Clin N Am 68 (2024) 319–335
https://doi.org/10.1016/j.cden.2023.09.006
0011-8532/24/© 2023 Elsevier Inc. All rights reserved.

Box 1	
Examples of malignant lesions of the oral region	
Primary carcinomas	Squamous cell carcinoma (90%)
	Mucoepidermoid carcinoma
	Acinic cell carcinoma
	Adenoid cystic carcinoma
	Adenocarcinoma
	Ameloblastic carcinoma
	Clear cell odontogenic carcinoma
Primary sarcomas	Osteosarcoma
	Chondrosarcoma
	Rhabdomyosarcoma
	Ewing sarcoma
	Malignant schwannoma
Metastases	Breast
	Lung
	Colon
	Prostate
Hematological malignancies	Leukemia
	Lymphoma
	Langerhans cell histiocytosis
	Multiple myeloma

widening of the mandibular canal with destruction of its cortical boundary.[2] **Table 1** presents a summary of the radiographic findings of oral malignancy.

Malignant lesions that invade the alveolar process may mimic periapical and periodontal inflammatory disease and are often misdiagnosed as such, resulting in a delay in diagnosis.[3,4] Therefore, dental professionals must be aware of the clinical and radiographic findings of different oral malignancies so that appropriate oncologic referrals for evaluation and diagnosis can be made promptly. A clinical judgment can be made based on the patient's complaint, history, clinical findings, pulp testing, and radiographs to determine the origin of symptoms.

Modern diagnostic imaging modalities play an essential role in evaluating malignant pathology of the oral region. These imaging modalities include computed tomography (CT), magnetic resonance imaging (MRI), and positron emission tomography (PET). The anatomic information provided by CT and MRI is invaluable in identifying and staging oral tumors, as well as in guiding intervention options for biopsy and definitive management.[1] Functional imaging using PET or PET-CT with [^{18}F] fluorodeoxyglucose may improve detection of recurrence in a surveillance setting.[5]

Squamous Cell Carcinoma Arising in the Oral Mucosa

Definition and clinical features
SCC accounts for more than 90% of all malignant neoplasms of the oral cavity and oropharynx.[6] SCC of the oral region is the sixth most common cause of cancer-related death in the Unites States.[7] Characteristically, oral SCC affects individuals older than 40 years of age with a history of tobacco and alcohol abuse. Men are affected two to three times as often as women. However, there is a disproportionate increase in the incidence of oral SCC (especially tongue) among young adults (especially women) without a history of significant tobacco or alcohol use.[8] Other risk factors for oral carcinoma include radiation exposure, betel nut chewing, poor oral

Table 1
Summary of radiographic findings of oral malignancy

Imaging Feature	Descriptor	Significance	Examples
Location	Mandible > maxilla Posterior region > anterior region	Presence of multifocal abnormalities in the jaws is suggestive of systemic disorder	Metastasis, multiple myeloma
Periphery	Ill-defined	Ragged and infiltrative periphery that lacks any cortication	SCC, lymphoma, metastasis
	Punched-out	Sharp boundary with no marginal bone reaction	Multiple myeloma, LCH
Internal structure	Radiolucent	"Moth-eaten" and permeative lytic lesion with trabecular remnants within the radiolucent area.	SCC, lymphoma, metastasis
	Mixed-density	Flocculent pattern of internal calcification	Chondrosarcoma
	Radiopaque	Patchy sclerotic bone formation	Osteosarcoma, metastasis (prostate and breast)
Effect on surrounding structures	"Floating teeth"	Extensive destruction of the supporting alveolar bone	SCC, metastasis, LCH
	Displacement of developing teeth in their crypts	Infiltration into the papilla of a developing tooth destroying the follicular cortex and displacing the developing tooth into the oral cavity	Leukemia, lymphoma, LCH
	"Spiked roots"	Tapered narrowing of the root	Osteosarcoma, chondrosarcoma
	Irregular widening of PDL space with loss of adjacent lamina dura	May simulate the appearance of periapical inflammatory disease	Metastasis, lymphoma
	Enlargement of a recent extraction socket	infiltration of the socket with malignant cells	SCC, osteosarcoma, metastasis
	Periosteal bone reaction	Periosteal bone formation that takes the form of laminations, spiculation, or Codman's triangle.	Osteosarcoma, LCH, metastasis (prostate)
	Irregular widening and destruction of the cortical borders of the neurovascular canals/foramina	Perineural tumor spread	SCC, adenoid cystic carcinoma

hygiene, human papillomavirus infection, candidal infection, tertiary syphilis, submucous fibrosis, and immunosuppression.[9]

The most affected sites for oral SCC are the floor of the mouth, the posterior lateral and ventral surfaces of the tongue, and soft palate.[10] Other less common sites of involvement include the retromolar trigone, buccal mucosa, gingiva, and hard palate.[7] Clinical staging for oral SCC is performed using the TNM (tumor, nodes, metastases) system that takes into account the tumor's size (thickness) and the presence of nodal and distant metastasis.[11]

Imaging features

The main imaging modalities for evaluation of oral SCCs are contrast-enhanced CT, MRI, and PET imaging.[1] CT is helpful in delineating the extent of disease and detecting subtle cortical bone erosion and periosteal reaction. SCCs typically appear as variably enhancing homogenous or heterogenous soft-tissue density lesions (**Figs. 1**A–C and **2**A–C). One disadvantage of CT in the oral region is image distortion caused by streak artifacts from dental restorations; however, visualization of an area can be improved by modifying scan angles to avoid the artifacts. In addition, a CT acquired while the cheeks are puffed out may separate opposed mucosal surfaces and improve visualization of mucosal lesions in the vestibule and retromolar trigone area (**Fig. 3**A and B).[12]

MRI enables better delineation of the lesion margins because of its superior soft-tissue contrast and its ability to image directly in the coronal and sagittal planes.

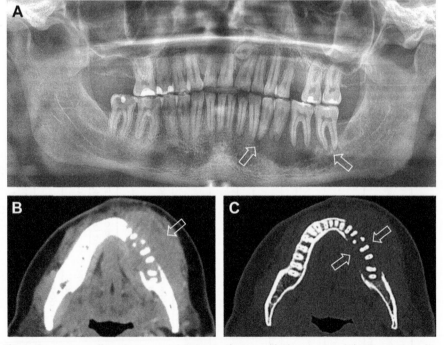

Fig. 1. Squamous cell carcinoma originating in the mandibular gingiva. (*A*) Panoramic radiograph shows bone destruction around the mandibular left premolars and molars, producing an appearance of teeth floating in space (*arrows*). (*B*) Axial contrast-enhanced CT (soft-tissue window setting) shows a mildly enhancing, destructive mass in the left buccal vestibule (*arrow*). (*C*) Axial CT (bone window setting) demonstrates destruction of the buccal and lingual cortical plates of the left mandible (*arrows*).

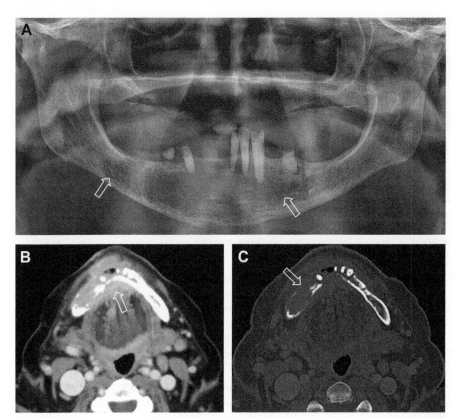

Fig. 2. Squamous cell carcinoma of the floor of mouth with secondary invasion of the mandible. (*A*) Panoramic image shows permeative destructive changes in the mandibular symphysis and body on the right. The areas of bone destruction blend imperceptibly with the adjacent normal bone (*arrows*). Also note the apical root resorption. (*B*) Axial contrast-enhanced CT image in soft-tissue window demonstrates an enhancing invasive lesion in the anterior floor of mouth (*arrow*). (*C*) Axial CT image in bone window demonstrates gross invasion of the mandible and cortical breakthrough on both sides (*arrow*).

SCC tends of have intermediate signal intensity equal to or lower than that of muscle on T1-weighted, high signal intensity on T2-weighted, and variable enhancement on post-contrast T1-weighted MR images.[13,14] MRI is the preferred modality for detection of perineural tumor spread and bone marrow invasion.[15] Combined PET-CT examination allows for characterization of both primary tumors and metastatic disease (**Fig. 4**)[5]

Most SCCs affecting the jaw originate in the gums (gingiva and alveolar mucosa) and secondarily invade the underlying bone.[14] Bone invasion is present in about 50% of gingiva carcinomas at the time of clinical presentation.[16] The first evidence of bone invasion may appear as irregular widening of the periodontal ligament space with loss of the adjacent lamina dura. Bone destruction soon becomes more profound, resulting in "floating teeth." The irregular and ill-defined regions of bone resorption may create a "moth-eaten" appearance. Remnants of trabecular bone within the radiolucent defect are seen infrequently. There may be a reactive peripheral sclerosis in the case of the presence of a secondary inflammatory disease. Perineural extension of SCC may result in irregular enlargement of the mandibular canal and mental

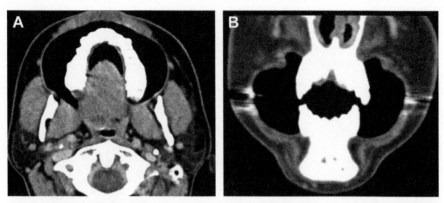

Fig. 3. Puffed-cheek technique. Axial (*A*) and coronal (*B*) reformatted contrast-enhanced CT images with the cheeks blown out to separate opposed mucosal surfaces and improve visualization of mucosal lesions in the vestibule and retromolar trigone. (*Courtesy of* Richard Wiggins, MD, Salt Lake City, UT)

foramen with loss of their cortical boundaries (**Fig. 5**A and B).[2] The destruction of the mandible may become so great as to cause a pathologic fracture. Some carcinomas of the jaw present an appearance in that the margins of bone destruction are moderately well-defined with no suggestion of infiltration.

Primary Intraosseous Squamous Cell Carcinoma

Definition and clinical features
Primary intraosseous SCC (PIOSCC) is a central jaw carcinoma arising from odontogenic epithelial remnants.[17] According to the World Health Organization classification

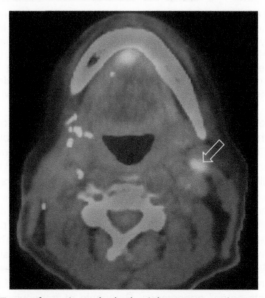

Fig. 4. Axial PET-CT scan of a patient who had a right tongue carcinoma treated with partial glossectomy, selective neck dissection, and chemoradiation therapy. On the 6-month surveillance scan, there is a left level IIB node that demonstrates high metabolic activity (*arrow*). Needle biopsy revealed metastatic carcinoma.

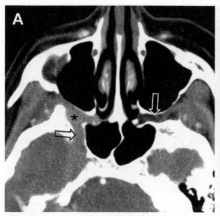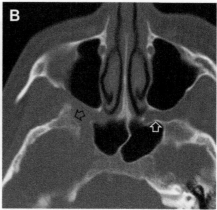

Fig. 5. Adenoid cystic carcinoma of the palate with perineural spread of tumor (PNS). (*A*) Axial contrast-enhanced soft-tissue window CT image demonstrates soft-tissue density tumor infiltrating and expanding the pterygopalatine fossa (PPF) (*asterisk*). Note the obliteration of the normal fat density within the PPF by tumor as compared with the normal left side (*white arrow*). Posteriorly, tumor is extending and widening the foramen rotundum into the cavernous sinus (*black arrow*) consistent with PNS. (*B*) Axial bone window CT image demonstrates asymmetric enlargement of the right PPF with erosive changes of its cortical margin (*black arrow*) as compared with the left side (*white arrow*). (*Courtesy of* Richard Wiggins, MD, Salt Lake City, UT)

published in 2005, PIOSCCs are classified into three subtypes: (1) a solid tumor that invades marrow spaces and induces osseous resorption, (2) SCC arising from the lining of an odontogenic cyst, and (3) SCC in association with other benign epithelial odontogenic tumors.

PIOSCC represents only 1% to 2% of all oral cavity carcinomas.[18] It occurs most commonly in middle-aged adults, with a mean age of 55 years at the time of diagnosis. Men are affected nearly twice as often as women. Most lesions occur in the posterior areas of the mandible, and maxillary lesions tend to occur in the anterior region.[19] Lesions can remain clinically silent until they reach an advanced stage. Patients may complain of pain, swelling, loosening of teeth, or paresthesia.

Imaging features
The solid variant of intraosseous carcinoma appears as a central ill-defined area of bone destruction with ragged margins. The irregular extension of the tumor may leave islands or strands of residual bone within the radiolucent defect. The radiographic findings of carcinoma arising in an odontogenic cyst may mimic those of any odontogenic cyst, but the periphery of the radiolucent defect is usually ill-defined and has an invasive characteristic commonly seen in malignant tumors (**Fig. 6**A–D). Late lesions are more obviously destructive.

Ameloblastic Carcinoma

Definition and clinical features
Ameloblastic carcinoma is a rare primary odontogenic malignancy that shows the histologic features of ameloblastoma with cellular atypia. It may arise de novo or, less commonly, from a preexisting ameloblastoma. About two-thirds of all reported cases have been found in the mandible, most often in the posterior areas. Men and women are affected with about equal frequency. It tends to occur in older patients, with most

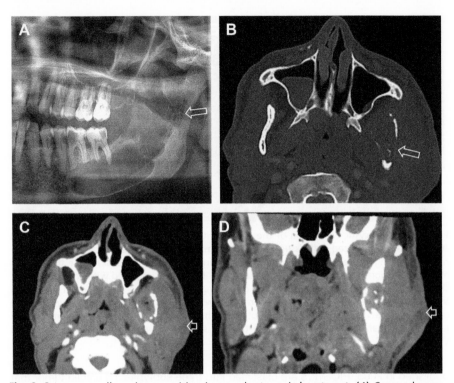

Fig. 6. Squamous cell carcinoma arising in an odontogenic keratocyst. (*A*) Cropped panoramic image shows a multilocular radiolucent lesion in the left mandibular body and ramus. Note the ill-defined, infiltrative periphery in the ramus (*arrow*). (*B*) Axial CT image (bone window) shows expansion and destruction of the outer cortices of ramus (*arrow*). Axial (*C*) and coronal (*D*) CT images (soft-tissue windows) show a large infiltrating mass that has eroded through the cortical bone and invaded the muscles of mastication and the overlying subcutaneous tissues and skin (*arrows*).

being older than 40 years of age. The tumor may exhibit an aggressive local behavior, with a propensity for regional and distant (lung) metastases.[20]

Imaging features
The radiographic presentation of ameloblastic carcinoma may be very similar to that of ameloblastoma. The lesion margins may be well-defined or poorly defined and infiltrative (**Fig. 7**A–C).

Osteosarcoma (Osteogenic Sarcoma)

Definition and clinical features
Osteosarcoma is a malignant tumor characterized by the formation of osteoid or immature bone. Osteosarcomas are rare in the jaws and account for 7% of all cases.[21] Patients with osteosarcoma of the jaws usually present in the fourth decade, approximately one decade later than patients with osteosarcoma of the long bones. The mandible and maxilla are affected with about equal frequency. In the mandible, the posterior body and ascending ramus are the most common sites; in the maxilla, the alveolar process and sinus floor are the sites of predilection. Patients typically present with a painful, rapidly growing mass. Loosening of teeth and paresthesia are common findings.[22]

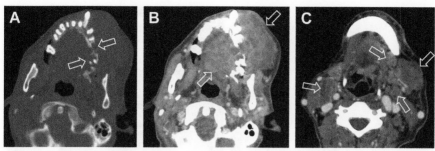

Fig. 7. Ameloblastic carcinoma. Axial contrast-enhanced CT images displayed in bone (*A*) and soft-tissue (*B*) window settings show a large, heterogeneously enhancing, infiltrative mass involving the left maxillary alveolus and extending into the cheek and soft palate (*arrows*). (*C*) Axial CT image at the level the inferior border of the mandible shows multiple bilateral necrotic metastatic lymph nodes in the submandibular and superior deep cervical lymph chains (*arrows*). (*Courtesy of* Ilson Sepúlveda, BDS, Concepción, Chile).

Imaging features

The radiographic appearance of osteosarcoma varies from totally radiolucent to mixed radiolucent and radiopaque to quite radiopaque. The periphery is usually ill-defined and indistinct. The lesion has a tendency to break through the cortical bone and stimulate the periosteum to produce linear bony spicules emanating from the bone surface in a "sunburst" pattern (**Fig. 8A–D**). In few cases, a triangular elevation of the periosteum at the periphery, referred to as Codman's triangle, may be observed.[22,23] Tumors in the alveolar process may, in early stages, infiltrate rapidly along the periodontal ligament space around teeth, resulting in irregular widening with destruction of the lamina dura.[24] This radiographic finding may be accompanied by local pain or tooth mobility and is of great importance in the early diagnosis of osteosarcoma. The roots of teeth may be resorbed into a "spiked" shape. A subtle but highly suggestive sign of osteosarcoma is the buildup of interproximal sclerotic bone beyond the normal height of alveolar bone. This finding has also been observed in chondrosarcoma.[25] In some instances, an osteosarcoma may have a radiographic pattern similar to that of a benign fibro-osseous lesion.[22,26] Cortical involvement and tumor calcification can be easily assessed by CT. However, the extent of intramedullary and extraosseous involvement may be seen better with MRI.[23]

Rhabdomyosarcoma

Definition and clinical features

Rhabdomyosarcoma is a malignant tumor of skeletal muscle phenotype. These tumors account for about 50% of soft-tissue sarcomas in children, with 40% of all cases occurring in the head and neck regions.[27] The most common sites are the orbit, nasopharynx, middle ear, sinonasal cavity, and masticator space (infratemporal fossa).[28,29] There are three histopathologic types of rhabdomyosarcoma: (1) embryonal, which is the most common type and predominates in younger children; (2) alveolar, which is the most aggressive type and more commonly seen in adolescents; and (3) pleomorphic, which occurs mainly in patients older than 40 years of age and primarily affects the extremities. There is an overall slight male predilection.[30] Symptoms depend on the site and size of the tumor and include nasal obstruction, epistaxis, rhinorrhea, proptosis, facial swelling, and recurrent otitis media.[31]

Imaging features

Rhabdomyosarcomas have density similar to that of muscle on unenhanced CT studies and are frequently associated with erosion and remodeling of the adjacent

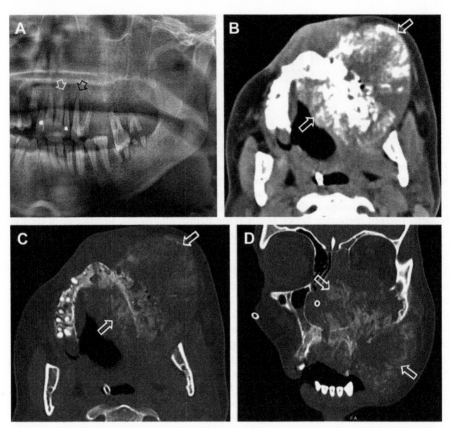

Fig. 8. Osteosarcoma of the maxilla. (*A*) Cropped panoramic image shows diffuse osteolytic and sclerotic changes involving the left maxilla and maxillary sinus. Note the "spiking" root resorption of the maxillary central incisors (*white arrow*) and widening of the periodontal ligament space around the left lateral incisor and canine (*black arrow*). (*B*) Axial CT image (soft-tissue window) shows a large, sclerotic, destructive mass with marked invasion of surrounding soft tissue (*arrows*). Axial (*C*) and coronal (*D*) CT images (bone windows) showing extensive bone destruction with tumor extension into the nasal and orbital region. Note the aggressive periosteal reaction caused by radiating mineralized tumor spicules (*arrows*).

bone (**Fig. 9**A, B). They are typically isointense or slightly hyperintense to muscle on T1-weighted images and hyperintense to muscle on T2-weighted images. There is diffuse but heterogenous enhancement on post-contrast CT and MR images.[32]

Metastatic Tumors to the Jaws

Definition and clinical features

Metastatic tumors are the second most common malignant neoplasms of the jaws after direct invasion from mucosal carcinomas.[33] Although metastasis to the jaw may arise from primary carcinomas of any anatomic site, the most frequent primary sites include, in order of decreasing incidence, the breast, lung, adrenal, kidney, colorectum, and prostate.[34] Most cases have been reported in middle-aged and older adults, with a mean age of 52 years.[35] The posterior segments of the jaws are more commonly affected, and the mandible is involved more commonly than the maxilla (a 5:1 ratio).[36]

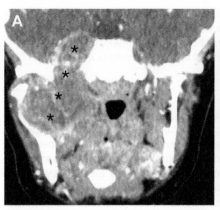
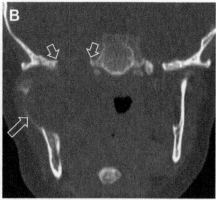

Fig. 9. Rhabdomyosarcoma in the masticator space/infratemporal fossa. (*A*) Coronal contrast-enhanced CT image demonstrates a heterogeneously enhancing, destructive mass involving the right masticator space/infratemporal fossa and extending through the skull base into the cranial cavity (*asterisks*). (*B*) Coronal CT imaging displayed in bone window settings demonstrates a large area of skull base destruction (*short arrows*) and erosion and lateral bowing of the ramus (*long arrow*). (*Courtesy of* Bernadette Koch, MD, Cincinnati, OH).

Bilateral involvement of the mandible occasionally occurs. Metastatic spread to the jaws is associated with a poor prognosis, and most patients die within 1 year.[37] Patients may be asymptomatic, or they may complain of pain, swelling, paresthesia, loosening of teeth, or a nonhealing extraction socket.[38]

Imaging features
Metastatic lesions usually appear as radiolucent defects with infiltrative or well-demarcated margins. Some lesions, particularly metastases from prostate and breast cancers, may stimulate new bone formation and present a radiopaque or mixed radiopaque–radiolucent appearance, often with a spiculated type of periosteal reaction (**Fig. 10**A and B). If the tumor is seeded in the alveolar process, it may cause destruction of the lamina dura and irregular widening of the periodontal ligament space around the involved teeth, mimicking periodontal and periapical inflammatory

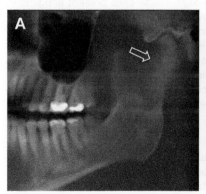
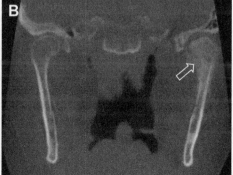

Fig. 10. Metastatic colon carcinoma to the mandibular condyle. Cropped reformatted panoramic (*A*) and coronal (*B*) cone-beam CT images demonstrate a sclerotic, destructive lesion of the left condyle, with a spiculated periosteal reaction along the adjacent cortices (*arrows*).

disease. Root resorption is rare. The sockets of teeth lost to metastatic disease may fail to heal or even increase in size.[35] On occasion, patients with jaw metastasis will have symptoms when conventional radiographs fail to demonstrate any changes. In such instances, bone scintigraphy with technetium usually reveals the lesion.

Lymphoma

Definition and clinical features

Lymphoma has been reported as the second most common malignancy of the extra-cranial head and neck after SCC.[39] It is typically classified as Hodgkin's lymphoma and non-Hodgkin's lymphoma. Both types of lymphoma occur in the head and neck. Hodgkin's lymphoma primarily presents as nodal disease, whereas non-Hodg-kin's lymphoma frequently involves extranodal sites, especially the Waldeyer's ring structures (adenoids, palatine tonsils, and lingual tonsils). Other primary sites include the parotid gland, palate, gingiva, buccal mucosa, orbit, and sinonasal cavity.[40] Most of the non-Hodgkin's lymphomas are B cell in origin. There is a male predominance, and the incidence increases with age and in immunocompromised patients. Epstein–Barr virus seems to be associated with lymphomas developing in the setting of immunosuppression.[41] Oral lymphoma often presents as a localized, boggy, non-tender swelling that may or may not be ulcerated.

Imaging features

The lesion typically appears as a fairly homogenous enhancing mass on CT and MRI. Cervical lymph node involvement is present in 80% of patients at presentation.[42] Un-like SCC and adenoid cystic carcinoma, perineural tumor spread of lymphoma is rare.[43] Lesions involving the maxilla often destroy the underlying bone, growing into the sinonasal cavity and orbital region (**Fig. 11**A–F). Lymphoma may infiltrate the peri-apical tissues and simulate periapical inflammatory disease. Another frequent radio-graphic presentation in the jaws is that of an ill-defined osteolytic lesion involving the alveolar bone, with margins suggestive of infiltration.[44] Some lesions stimulate a periosteal reaction that may take the form of a laminated or spiculated pattern.

Langerhans Cell Histiocytosis

Definition and clinical features

Langerhans cell histiocytosis (LCH) is a spectrum of diseases caused by neoplastic clonal proliferation of Langerhans cells or their precursors. Langerhans cells are den-dritic mononuclear cells normally found in the skin. These cells present antigens to lymph nodes for further processing by the immune system.[45]

Although LCH occurs across a wide age range, most of the affected patients are younger than 15 years of age.[46] Men are affected more often than women, and whites are affected more frequently than blacks. Bone lesions are the most common clinical presentation. Lesions can be solitary or multiple with or without visceral involvement. Most lesions occur in the cranial vault, mandible, ribs, and vertebrae.[47] Jaw involve-ment is more common in the mandible than the maxilla. The disease may cause local pain, tenderness, and swelling.

Imaging features

Early lesions appear as poorly defined lytic areas with laminated periosteal bone reac-tion. More mature lesions may show sclerotic margins and expanded remodeled appearance due to the laminated periosteal bone formation (**Fig. 12**A and B). The lesion often has a beveled edge or double contour resulting from uneven destruction of the outer cortical plates.[47] The destructive process starts in the midroot region and extends in a circular shape to involve the crestal portion of the alveolar process, which

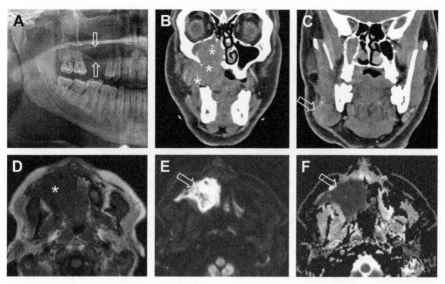

Fig. 11. Lymphoma (non-Hodgkin's). (*A*) Cropped panoramic image demonstrates ill-defined bone destruction in the periapical area of the right maxillary canine and first premolar. Note the effacement of the alveolar crest and hard palate (*arrows*). (*B*) Coronal contrast-enhanced CT image shows a homogenously enhancing destructive mass involving the right maxillary sinus and nasal cavity (*asterisks*). (*C*) Coronal contrast-enhanced CT image shows a large right level IB node that is homogenous and well delineated (*arrow*). (*D*) Axial T1-weighted MR image shows a homogenous mass with intermediate signal intensity (*asterisk*). (*E*) Diffusion-weighted image (DWI) and (*F*) apparent diffusion coefficient (ADC) map from MR imaging show restricted diffusion with high signal on the DWI (*arrow* in *E*) and low signal on the ADC map (*arrow* in *F*), suggesting a lesion with high cellularity.

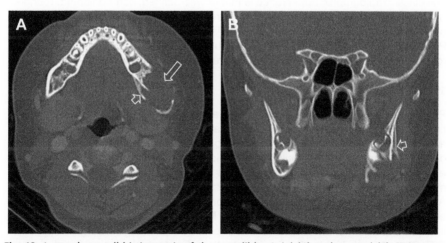

Fig. 12. Langerhans cell histiocytosis of the mandible. Axial (*A*) and coronal (*B*) CT images (bone window setting) demonstrate an aggressive lytic lesion in the left posterior mandible. The lesion has caused destruction of the outer cortical bone (*long arrow*). Note the laminated periosteal bone formation, which has caused an "expanded" appearance (*short arrows*). (*Courtesy of* Bernadette Koch, MD, Cincinnati, OH)

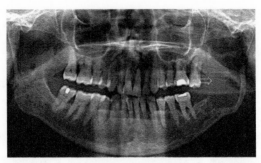

Fig. 13. Multiple myeloma. Panoramic image shows a large, well-defined, destructive lesion in the left ramus of the mandible (*arrow*). Also note the punched-out, rounded, lytic lesions scattered throughout the mandible and malar bone.

may give the lesion a "scooped-out" appearance.[2] Lesions tend to destroy the supporting alveolar bone, which produces the appearance of "floating teeth."

Multiple Myeloma

Definition and clinical features
Multiple myeloma is a malignant monoclonal proliferation of plasma cells, which is characterized by multicentric or diffuse bone involvement. The disease most frequently affects adults older than 40 years of age, with a mean age of 60 years and a slight male predilection. Patients may complaint of bone pain, fatigue, weight loss, fever, and anemia.[48] Increased susceptibility to infection is common as a result of neutropenia. Metastatic calcification of the soft tissues may occur as a result of hypercalcemia. Plasmacytoma is the solitary counterpart of multiple myeloma. The jaws are affected in 20% to 30% of cases.[49] The lesions are more common in the mandible than in the maxilla and are most often seen in the posterior body, ramus, and condyle.

Imaging features
The classic radiographic appearance is that of well-defined, non-corticated, rounded, "punched-out" lytic lesions with no bone reaction in the immediately surrounding bone.[50] Adjacent lesions may coalesce into larger areas of bone destruction (**Fig. 13**). Pathologic fracture of the mandible may occur. Lesions do not characteristically cause root resorption. There is no periosteal bone reaction in most cases.

SUMMARY

Primary and metastatic malignancies may affect the jaws and mimic periapical inflammatory disease. Clinicians should be aware of the potential for this problem, and patients should be referred for appropriate evaluation and diagnosis. In such cases, a normal response to pulp testing indicates a nonodontogenic lesion. A careful evaluation of radiographs is an integral part of the examination protocol. Alternative methods, such as cone-beam CT, may provide important diagnostic information. Advanced imaging modalities play an important role in the preoperative evaluation and staging of oral region cancers. CT and MRI are invaluable in demonstrating the location and extent of the tumor, which is important in planning the surgical approach. PET-CT imaging is highly effective in detection of metastasis and recurrent disease.

DISCLOSURE

The authors declare that they have no conflict of interest.

REFERENCES

1. Weber AL, Romo L, Hashmi S. Malignant tumors of the oral cavity and oropharynx: clinical, pathologic, and radiologic evaluation. Neuroimaging Clin N Am 2003;13: 443–64.
2. White S, Pharoah M. Malignant diseases. In: White S, Pharoah M, editors. Oral radiology: principles & interpretation. 7th edition. St Louis (MO): Elsevier; 2014. p. 563–81.
3. Pereira DL, Fernandes DT, Santos-Silva AR, et al. Intraosseous non-Hodgkin lymphoma mimicking a periapical lesion. J Endod 2015;41(10):1738–42.
4. Selden HS, Manhoff DT, Hatges NA, et al. Metastatic carcinoma to the mandible that mimicked pulpal/periodontal disease. J Endod 1998;24(4):267–70.
5. Agarwal V, Branstetter BF 4th, Johnson JT. Indications for PET/CT in the head and neck. Otolaryngol Clin North Am 2008;41(1):23–49.
6. Kirsch C. Oral cavity cancer. Top Magn Reson Imaging 2007;18:269–80.
7. Kademani D. Oral cancer. Mayo Clin Proc 2007;82:878–87.
8. Bleyer A. Cancer of the oral cavity and pharynx in young females: increasing incidence, role of human papilloma virus, and lack of survival improvement. Semin Oncol 2009;36:451–9.
9. Neville BW, Damm DD, Allen CM. Epithelial pathology. In: Neville BW, Damm DD, Allen CM, Bouquot JE, editors. Oral and maxillofacial pathology. 3rd edition. Philadelphia, PA: Saunders; 2008. p. 362–452.
10. Mashberg A, Samit A. Early diagnosis of asymptomatic oral and oropharyngeal squamous cancers. CA Cancer J Clin 1995;45:328–51.
11. Edge SB, American Joint Committee on Cancer. AJCC cancer staging manual. 7th Edition. New York: Springer; 2010.
12. Weissman JL, Carrau RL. "Puffed-cheek" CT improves evaluation of the oral cavity. AJNR Am J Neuroradiol 2001;22:741–4.
13. Beil CM, Keberle M. Oral and oropharyngeal tumors. Eur J Radiol 2008;66: 448–59.
14. Sigal R, Zagdanski AM, Schwaab G, et al. CT and MR imaging of squamous cell carcinoma of the tongue and floor of the mouth. Radiographics 1996;16:787–810.
15. Mao YP, Liang SB, Liu LZ, et al. The N staging system in nasopharyngeal carcinoma with radiation therapy oncology group guidelines for lymph node levels based on magnetic resonance imaging. Clin Cancer Res 2008;14:7497–503.
16. Gomez D, Faucher A, Picot V, et al. Outcome of squamous cell celrcinoma of the gingiva: a follow-up study of 83 cases. J Cranio-Maxillo-Fac Surg 2000;28(6): 331–5.
17. Barnes L. Pathology and genetics of head and neck tumours. Lyon: IARC Press; 2005.
18. Bodner L, Manor E, Shear M, et al. Primary intraosseous squamous cell carcinoma arising in an odontogenic cyst: a clinicopathologic analysis of 116 reported cases. J Oral Pathol Med 2011;40(10):733–8.
19. de Morais EF, Carlan LM, de Farias Morais HG, et al. Primary intraosseous squamous cell carcinoma involving the jaw bones: a systematic review and update. Head Neck Pathol 2021;15(2):608–16.
20. Cho BH, Jung YH, Hwang JJ. Ameloblastic carcinoma of the mandible: A case report. Imaging Sci Dent 2020;50(4):359–63.
21. Weber AL, Bui C, Kaneda T. Malignant tumors of the mandible and maxilla. Neuroimaging Clin N Am 2003;13(3):509–24.

22. Nakayama E, Sugiura K, Ishibashi H, et al. The clinical and diagnostic imaging findings of osteosarcoma of the jaw. Dentomaxillofac Radiol 2005;34(3):182–8.

23. Luo Z, Chen W, Shen X, et al. Head and neck osteosarcoma: CT and MR imaging features. Dentomaxillofac Radiol 2020;49(2):20190202.

24. Garrington GE, Scofield HH, Cornyn J, et al. Osteosarcoma of the jaws. Analysis of 56 cases. Cancer 1967;20(3):377–91.

25. Garrington GE, Collett WK. Chondrosarcoma. II. Chondrosarcoma of the jaws: analysis of 37 cases. J Oral Pathol 1988;17(1):12–20.

26. Wang S, Shi H, Yu Q. Osteosarcoma of the jaws: demographic and CT imaging features. Dentomaxillofac Radiol 2012;41(1):37–42.

27. Paulino AC, Okcu MF. Rhabdomyosarcoma. Curr Probl Cancer 2008;32:7–34.

28. Sturgis EM, Potter BO. Sarcomas of the head and neck region. Curr Opin Oncol 2003;15:239–52.

29. Darwish C, Shim T, Sparks AD, et al. Pediatric head and neck rhabdomyosarcoma: An analysis of treatment and survival in the United States (1975-2016). Int J Pediatr Otorhinolaryngol 2020;139:110403.

30. Anderson GJ, Tom LW, Womer RB, et al. Rhabdomyosarcoma of the head and neck in children. Arch Otolaryngol Head Neck Surg 1990;116(4):428–31.

31. Herrmann BW, Sotelo-Avila C, Eisenbeis JF. Pediatric sinonasal rhabdomyosarcoma: three cases and a review of the literature. Am J Otolaryngol 2003;24:174–80.

32. Kim EE, Valenzuela RF, Kumar AJ, et al. Imaging and clinical spectrum of rhabdomyosarcoma in children. Clin Imaging 2000;24:257–62.

33. Hirshberg A, Buchner A. Metastatic tumours to the oral region. An overview. Eur J Cancer B Oral Oncol 1995;31B(6):355–60.

34. Hirshberg A, Leibovich P, Buchner A. Metastatic tumors to the jawbones: analysis of 390 cases. J Oral Pathol Med 1994;23(8):337–41.

35. Hirshberg A, Shnaiderman-Shapiro A, Kaplan I, et al. Metastatic tumours to the oral cavity - pathogenesis and analysis of 673 cases. Oral Oncol 2008;44(8):743–52.

36. D'Silva NJ, Summerlin DJ, Cordell KG, et al. Metastatic tumors in the jaws: a retrospective study of 114 cases. J Am Dent Assoc 2006;137(12):1667–72.

37. Hirshberg A, Berger R, Allon I, et al. Metastatic tumors to the jaws and mouth. Head Neck Pathol 2014;8(4):463–74.

38. Hirshberg A, Leibovich P, Horowitz I, et al. Metastatic tumors to postextraction sites. J Oral Maxillofac Surg 1993;51:1334–7.

39. Epstein JB, Epstein JD, Le ND, et al. Characteristics of oral and paraoral malignant lymphoma: a population-based review of 361 cases. Oral Surg Oral Med Oral Pathol Oral Radiol Endod 2001;92:519–25.

40. Mendenhall N. Lymphomas and related diseases presenting in the head and neck. In: Million R, Cassisi N, editors. Management of head and neck cancer: a multidisciplinary approach. Philadelphia: JB Lippincott; 1994. p. 857–78.

41. Landgren O, Caporaso NE. New aspects in descriptive, etiologic, and molecular epidemiology of Hodgkin's lymphoma. Hematol Oncol Clin North Am 2007;21:825–40.

42. Wong DS, Fuller LM, Butler JJ, et al. Extranodal non-Hodgkin's lymphomas of the head and neck. Am J Roentgenol Radium Ther Nucl Med 1975;123:471–81.

43. Laine FJ, Braun IF, Jensen ME, et al. Perineural tumor extension through the foramen ovale: evaluation with MR imaging. Radiology 1990;174:65–71.

44. Pazoki A, Jansisyanont P, Ord RA. Primary non-Hodgkin's lymphoma of the jaws: Report of 4 cases and review of the literature. J Oral Maxillofac Surg 2003;61(1):112–7.

45. Chu T, Jaffe R. The normal Langerhans cell and the LCH cell. Br J Cancer Suppl 1994;23:S4–10.

46. Nicholson HS, Egeler RM, Nesbit ME. The epidemiology of Langerhans cell histiocytosis. Hematol Oncol Clin North Am 1998;12(2):379–84.

47. Stull MA, Kransdorf MJ, Devaney KO. Langerhans cell histiocytosis of bone. Radiographics 1992;12(4):801–23.

48. Lae ME, Vencio EF, Inwards CY, et al. Myeloma of the jaw bones: a clinicopathologic study of 33 cases. Head Neck 2003;25(5):373–81.

49. Lu SY, Ma MC, Wang MC, et al. The status of jaw lesions and medication-related osteonecrosis of jaw in patients with multiple myeloma. J Formos Med Assoc 2021;120(11):1967–76.

50. Witt C, Borges AC, Klein K, et al. Radiographic manifestations of multiple myeloma in the mandible: a retrospective study of 77 patients. J Oral Maxillofac Surg 1997;55(5):450–3.

Imaging of the Sinonasal Cavities

Ilson Sepúlveda A, DDS, MSc[a,b,*], Francisco Rivas-Rodriguez, MD[c],
Aristides A. Capizzano, MD[c]

KEYWORDS

- Sinonasal • Cavities • Imaging • Inflammatory • Tumor • CT • MRI

KEY POINTS

- Inflammatory polyps are the most common expansile sinonasal lesions encountered in clinical practice.
- Computed tomography (CT) and MRI play a complementary role in the evaluation of sinonasal pathologic condition.
- Imaging characteristics that are suggestive of benignity include well-defined margins, bone remodeling or sclerosis, involvement of a single paranasal sinus, homogeneity, low attenuation on CT, high T2 signal intensity, and high apparent diffusion coefficient (ADC) values on MR imaging.
- Imaging characteristics that are suggestive of malignancy include irregular margins, erosion and bone fragmentation, extension beyond the sinus walls, high attenuation on CT, low T2 signal intensity, and low ADC values on MR imaging.
- Contrast-enhanced MR imaging is useful in detecting perineural tumor spread and dural invasion.

INTRODUCTION

Anatomically, the sinonasal cavities are composed of bone and cartilage lined by respiratory columnar epithelium and are located between the orbital cavity and the oral cavity. They are also close to the frontal cortex through the cribriform lamina of the ethmoid and are connected to the endocranium through vessels, lymphatic channels, and nerves. The olfactory mucosa is innervated by the olfactory nerve; the sensory innervation of the ethmoid sinus, sphenoid sinus, lateral wall of the nasal cavity, and the anterior part of the nasal septum is supplied by the ophthalmic nerve (V1); and

[a] Finis Terrae University School of Dentistry, Santiago, Chile; [b] Radiology Department, ENT-Head&Neck Surgery and Maxillofacial Services, General Hospital of Concepción, San Martín Av. N° 1436, Concepción, Chile; [c] Division of Neuroradiology, University of Michigan, 1500 East Medical Center Dr, B2A205, Ann Arbor, MI 48109-5302, USA
* Corresponding author. ENT-Head&Neck Surgery and Maxillofacial Services, General Hospital of Concepción, San Martín Av. n° 1436 Concepción, Chile.
E-mail address: isepulvedaa@uft.edu

the sensory innervation of the maxillary sinus is supplied by the maxillary nerve (V2). The components of the anterior sinonasal region drain to the submandibular lymph nodes (level II) while the posterior components drain to the retropharyngeal lymph nodes.[1–3]

The histologic diversity of neoplasms in the sinonasal cavities is surprisingly high, considering that their apparent content is air and a thin mucosal lining. However, this region has one of the widest ranges of neoplasms among all anatomic sites in the head and neck, with more than 70 types of tumors described, which may be of epithelial, mesenchymal, lymphoid, or melanocytic origin (**Table 1**). Epithelial and mesenchymal tumors can be benign or malignant, whereas lymphoid and melanocytic tumors of the sinonasal region are usually malignant.

Inflammatory polyps are the most common expansile sinonasal lesions encountered in clinical practice. However, the true differentiation between benign and malignant lesions is difficult in all imaging modalities because among other characteristics, these entities present with very similar frequencies.

In the case of malignant tumors of the sinonasal cavities, these are rare and aggressive, representing 1% of all malignant tumors and 3% of all malignant neoplasms of the upper autodigestive tract being more common in men than in women (1.7:1) and occurring more commonly between the fourth and sixth decade of life.[4,5] The origin and histologic type vary in the different series, with squamous cell carcinoma (SCC) predominating, being observed in almost 70% of the cases in the maxillary sinus.[6] Other subtypes of malignant tumors such as adenocarcinoma, minor salivary gland carcinoma, undifferentiated carcinoma, neuroendocrine carcinoma, and nonepithelial malignant tumors such as sarcomas, lymphomas, plasmacytomas, olfactory neuroblastomas, and melanomas are considerably less common. It is necessary to mention that the incidence of lymphonodal metastasis in maxillary sinus carcinomas is low, less than 15%, but if present, it has a worse prognosis.

DIAGNOSTIC IMAGING

In the imaging evaluation, the objective is to determine whether the tumor in question is benign or malignant. Well-defined margins, bone remodeling or sclerosis, involvement of a single paranasal sinus, homogeneity, low attenuation on computed tomography (CT), and high signal intensity at long relaxation times on MRI are imaging characteristics suggestive of benignity. However, irregular margins, erosion and bone fragmentation, extension beyond the sinus walls, high attenuation on CT, and hypointense signal in long relaxation times on MRI are imaging characteristics that generate suspicion of a malignant process.[4,6–8]

For an optimal CT evaluation, it is necessary to perform acquisitions with slice thickness less than 1 mm and to perform multiplanar reconstructions. Key areas for CT evaluation are the bony walls of the orbital cavity, cribriform plate, ethmoidal fovea, posterior wall of the maxillary sinus, pterygopalatine fossa, pterygoid process, sphenoidal sinus, and posterior wall of the frontal sinus.[9,10]

Particularly in the case of sinonasal malignant neoplasms, the main objective is to determine their extension, including the identification of the primary tumor focus, sites of invasion (eg, skull base, orbit, brain, and vascular structures), mass effect on critical structures, evidence of perineural spread, and the presence or absence of lymphadenopathy.[11–14]

CT and MRI play a complementary role in the evaluation of sinonasal malignant neoplasms. CT is highly effective in the evaluation and definition of margins and patterns of bone infiltration and invasion, as well as in the determination of intralesional

Table 1
Classification of tumors and tumor-like lesions of the sinonasal cavities

Origin	Type
Epithelial	Schneiderian papillomas (fungiform, inverted, and oncocytic) SCC Adenocarcinoma Undifferentiated carcinoma
Salivary gland	Pleomorphic adenoma Adenoid cystic carcinoma Mucoepidermoid carcinoma
Neuroectodermal	Schwannoma Meningioma Olfactory neuroblastoma Malignant schwannoma Neuroendocrine carcinoma Melanoma
Soft tissue	Hemangioma Angiofibroma Hemangiopericytoma Hemangiosarcoma Rhabdomyosarcoma Fibrous histiocytoma
Bone, cartilaginous, and odontogenic tissue	Osteoma Ossifying fibroma Fibrous dysplasia Osteosarcoma Chondrosarcoma Ewing sarcoma Odontogenic keratocyst Ameloblastoma
Hematopoietic	Plasmacytoma Lymphoma Langerhans cell histiocytosis
Metastatic	Kidney Lung Breast Gastrointestinal tract Others
Developmental	Encephalocele Hamartoma Dermoid/epidermoid Teratoma
Miscellaneous	Inflammatory polyps Fungal infections Wegener granulomatosis Retention cyst Mucocele

calcifications. The use of water-soluble, nonionic intravenous contrast is decisive for the identification of the tumor vascular pattern.[2,4,15] As for MRI, this imaging modality allows us to distinguish the neoplasm from inflammatory changes and postobstructive secretions (T2 and fluid-attenuated inversion recovery sequences). It also allows us to demonstrate more clearly the invasion of the periorbital fat (fat-saturated and short tau inversion recovery [STIR] sequences), tumor invasion to the skull base, identifying dural infiltration, infiltration of the cavernous sinus, differentiation between tumor and muscle in the infratemporal fossa and masticator space, and separation of the tumor from critical neurovascular structures such as the optic nerve, internal carotid artery, and cavernous sinus (T1 and T2 sequences). Malignant neoplasms tend to show nonspecific signal intensities: hyperintense on T2 sequence and hypointense on T1 sequence.[11,16]

Lesions with a low apparent diffusion coefficient (ADC) and marked diffusion restriction indicate hypercellularity, abscess, or hemorrhage; however, lesions with a high ADC represent hypocellularity, mucus, cartilage, or fluid. Therefore, malignant sinonasal lesions present significantly lower ADC values than benign lesions. Intravenous gadolinium contrast is useful in detecting perineural tumor spread and dural invasion, with a sensitivity of 100% and a specificity of 95%.[15,17] Perineural tumor spread can be seen as enlargement and enhancement of the nerve, widening of the neural foramen, and obliteration of the normal perineural fat at the skull base foramina. Dural thickening greater than 5 mm or the presence of dural enhancing foci indicates meningeal invasion. Tumors commonly associated with perineural spread include SCC, adenoid cystic carcinoma, mucoepidermoid carcinoma, melanoma, and lymphoma.[11]

INFLAMMATORY DISEASES
Rhinoliths

Rhinoliths occur within the nasal fossae and are the result of deposition of mineral salts around a nidus, which eventually leads to formation of a stone. They are usually located in the floor of the nasal cavity under the inferior turbinate. Clinically they produce nasal obstruction and unilateral purulent rhinorrhea, epistaxis, and pain. On CT, they seem as hyperdense bodies of irregular morphology associated with chronic inflammation of the nasal mucosa (**Fig. 1**A–C). Antroliths are similar calcifications but are found within the maxillary sinuses.[18–22]

Acute Rhinosinusitis

Acute rhinosinusitis (ARS) is a consequence of an upper respiratory tract infection. It is usually a self-limiting disease but severe complications leading to life-threatening situations have been described. CT of sinonasal region is indicated for cases of ARS that are associated with symptoms such as headache, facial enlargement, proptosis, and paralysis of one or more cranial nerves.[14,23,24] CT and MRI include nonspecific mucosal thickening within the ostiomeatal and/or sinus complex,

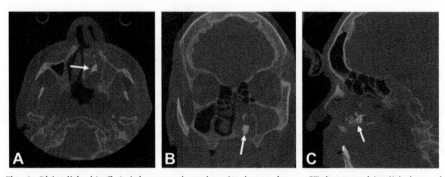

Fig. 1. Rhinolith. (*A–C*) Axial, coronal, and sagittal cone-beam CT shows a rhinolith (*arrow*) associated with complete opacification of the left nasal cavity and maxillary sinus.

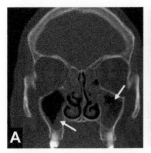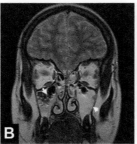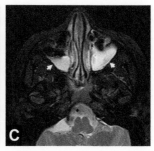

Fig. 2. ARS. (*A*) Coronal CT image shows mucosal thickening in both maxillary sinuses (*arrows*). Note the bubbly, frothy secretions in the left sinus. Coronal T2-weighted (*B*) and axial STIR (*C*) MR images demonstrate hyperintense postobstructive fluid, air collections, and obliteration of both maxillary sinuses (*arrowhead*).

submucosal edema, air-fluid levels, and sinus secretions associated with airborne collections (**Fig. 2**A–C).[1,25]

Complications of ARS can be classified as orbital, intracranial, or osseous. Orbital involvement includes preseptal edema or inflammation (periorbital cellulitis), postseptal orbital cellulitis, subperiosteal abscess, and orbital abscess. Intracranial complications include phlegmonous inflammation (eg, meningitis, cerebritis), abscess formation (epidural, subdural, or intracerebral), and cavernous sinus thrombosis (**Fig. 3**A–C).[3,16,26]

Chronic Rhinosinusitis

Chronic rhinosinusitis with or without nasal polyps is an inflammatory disorder involving the sinonasal cavities. On CT, it is characterized by uniform or polypoid thickening of the Schneiderian mucosa and intrasinusal calcifications associated with sclerosis of the sinus bony walls (**Fig. 4**A–C). This sclerotic bone corresponds to a reactive process and reflects the chronic nature of the disease.[23,25,27–30]

Non-invasive Fungal Rhinosinusitis

Noninvasive fungal rhinosinusitis ("fungus ball" or mycetoma) is the collection of fungal debris usually within a single paranasal sinus, with the maxillary sinus and sphenoid sinus being the most affected. On noncontrast CT, "calcifications" and sclerosis of

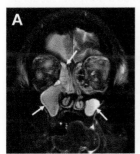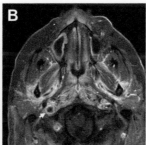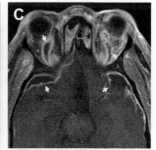

Fig. 3. Complicated ARS. (*A*) Coronal STIR image shows hyperintense mucosal thickening in the right maxillary sinus and ethmoid cells as well as postobstructive fluid and mucus retention cyst in the left maxillary sinus (*arrows*). (*B* and *C*) Axial fat-saturated post–contrast-enhanced T1-weighted images showing right internal jugular vein and bilateral superior ophthalmic vein thrombosis, and intracranial abscess (*arrowheads*).

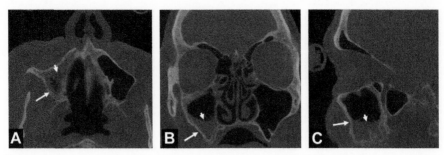

Fig. 4. Chronic rhinosinusitis. (*A–C*) Axial, coronal, and sagittal cone-beam CT images showing mucosal thickening in the right maxillary sinus, with postobstructive fluid level (*arrowheads*) and peripheral thickening of the antral bony walls (*arrows*).

the inner sinus wall are the most prevalent features for noninvasive fungal rhinosinusitis (**Fig. 5**A–C). To be more precise, the "calcifications" should be referred to as hyperdensities because they represent dense conglomerates of fungal hyphae and traces of metallic elements in the fungus. In the case of the mucosa, it is often less dense (hypoattenuating). Sclerosis and thickening are the most common findings at the bone level, followed by erosion (pressure necrosis) and remodeling. On contrast-enhanced CT, there is enhancement of the thickened mucosa along the sinus wall.[1,14,24,29,31,32]

Odontogenic Sinusitis

Odontogenic sinusitis occurs when the integrity of the Schneiderian membrane is compromised by odontogenic causes. CT is the imaging study of choice; however, radiologists may miss odontogenic causes of maxillary sinusitis in up to 60% of cases. The key imaging finding that suggests odontogenic cause of maxillary sinusitis is a hypodense apical lesion related to a posterior tooth. Potential iatrogenic causes for odontogenic sinusitis include oroantral communication, orthognathic surgery, sinus floor elevation procedures before dental implant placement, and foreign bodies such as root fragments and endodontic filling materials (**Fig. 6**A–C).[33–36]

Antrochoanal Polyp

The antrochoanal polyp is typically a unilateral, benign polypoid lesion that mainly affects boys and young adult men.[37] On CT, it typically seems as a polypoid, isodense,

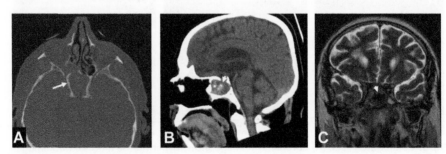

Fig. 5. Noninvasive fungal sinusitis. (*A*) Axial CT bone window image shows complete opacification of the sphenoid sinus with peripheral bony sclerosis (*arrow*). (*B*) Sagittal CT soft-tissue window shows hyperdense material within the sinus (*arrowhead*). (*C*) Coronal T2-weighted MR image shows hypointense signal of calcified material (*arrowhead*).

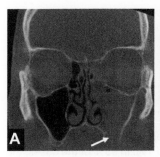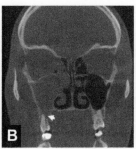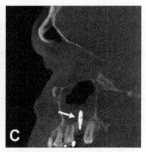

Fig. 6. Odontogenic rhinosinusitis. (*A*) Coronal cone-beam CT image shows complete opacification and oroantral fistula in the left maxillary sinus (*arrow*). (*B*) Coronal cone-beam CT image shows complete opacification of right maxillary sinus. Note the periapical lucency secondary to vertical dental fracture (*arrowhead*). (*C*) Sagittal cone-beam CT image shows generalized mucosal thickening associated with ectopic placement of the existing dental implant with sinus perforation and extension into the sinus cavity (*arrow*).

homogeneous mass, which completely occupies the maxillary sinus and middle meatus and extends toward the ipsilateral choana, without signs of expansion or bony erosion (**Fig. 7**A–C). There is no enhancement after the use of intravenous contrast.[2,38–40] Differential diagnosis includes conditions such as angiofibroma, mucocele, fungal allergic rhinosinusitis, inverted papilloma, olfactory neuroblastoma, and meningoencephalocele.[41]

Mucocele

Mucocele is a slow-growing, locally aggressive retention cyst. They are usually unilateral and affect the fronto-ethmoidal complex (60%–80%), followed by the maxillary sinus (10%) and the posterior ethmoid and sphenoid sinus (6%–11%). On CT, it seems as a smoothly expansile, homogeneous, isodense mass, with thinning and remodeling of the bony walls of the sinonasal cavity.[1,42–45] After administration of a contrast medium with CT, thin peripheral enhancement of the lesion is seen. On MRI, the signal intensity of mucocele varies depending on the protein content of the contained secretions and the presence or absence of secondary infection. A mucocele with a low protein content is hypointense on T1-weighted images and hyperintense on T2-weighted images. However, as time passes and the protein content increases, mucocele

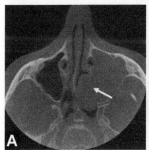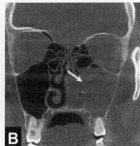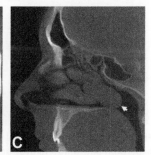

Fig. 7. Antrochoanal polyp. (*A* and *B*) Axial and coronal cone-beam CT showing complete opacification of the left maxillary sinus and polypoid mass at the level of the middle meatus with extension to the ipsilateral nasal cavity (*arrows*). (*C*) Sagittal cone-beam CT showing polypoid mass into the posterior choana (*arrowhead*).

changes its signal intensity, being hyperintense on T1-weighted images and hypointense on T2-weighted images (**Fig. 8**A–C). In all cases, on contrast-enhanced T1-weighted images, linear peripheral enhancement may be observed, without enhancement of the mucocele content.[46–48]

BENIGN NEOPLASMS
Bone and Fibro-Osseous Tumors

Osteomas
Osteomas are slow-growing, benign, bone-forming neoplasms. The incidence of osteoma in the sinonasal cavity varies between 0.43% and 1%. In 95% of the cases, the osteoma is located in the fronto-ethmoidal region.[4] On CT, it seems as a well-circumscribed, uniformly hyperdense mass with or without internal trabecular structure, depending on its histologic type. On MRI, the signal intensity is hypointense on T1-weighted and T2-weighted sequences (**Fig. 9**A–C). No enhancement is visualized after intravenous contrast administration, due to the high density of the lesion.[8,9]

Fibrous dysplasia
Fibrous dysplasia is a disorder of unknown origin where normal bone is replaced by fibrous tissue, bone metaplasia, and poorly calcified bone neoformation. It represents 2.5% of all bone lesions and 7% of benign bone tumors. It has 3 forms of clinical presentation: monostotic (70%), polyostotic (30%), and McCune-Albright syndrome (3%). On CT, it may seem as an expansile, homogeneous, hyperdense lesion with a characteristic "ground-glass" pattern (**Fig. 10**A–C). The relationship between the amount of fibrous tissue and the rate of bone apposition determines 3 patterns of presentation: pagetoid (56%), sclerotic (23%), and cystic (21%). The pagetoid type is characterized by areas of bony expansion associated with a mixture of sclerotic and cystic areas.[4,8,9]

Ossifying fibroma
Ossifying fibroma is a benign neoplasm consisting of fibrous tissue that contains various amounts of mineralized material. On CT, ossifying fibroma may seem as a well-defined, unilocular, expansile, hypodense lesion, with a variable amount of internal calcifications (**Fig. 11**A–C). After the use of intravenous contrast, it may show a slight enhancement at the level of its soft tissue component. The differential diagnosis

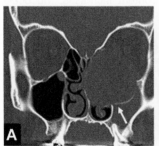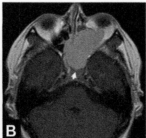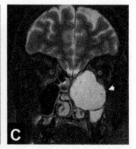

Fig. 8. Mucocele. (*A*) Coronal CT bone window shows a hypoattenuating mass causing expansion and thinning/destruction of the bony walls of the left maxillary sinus and orbital cavity (*arrow*). (*B*) Axial T1-weighted MRI sequence shows a moderately hyperintense lesion suggestive of high protein content (*arrowhead*). (*C*) Coronal STIR image shows a hyperintense cystic lesion associated with postobstructive secretions in ipsilateral maxillary sinus (*arrowhead*).

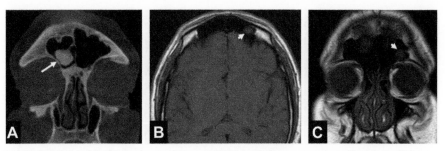

Fig. 9. Osteoma. (*A*) Coronal cone-beam CT image shows a round, uniformly radiopaque mass in the right frontal sinus (*arrow*). (*B* and *C*) Axial and coronal T1-weighted MRI on another patient show a hypointense mass in the left frontal sinus (*arrowhead*).

of ossifying fibroma should include fibrous dysplasia, solitary fibrous tumor, and osteosarcoma.[4,49–52]

Epithelial Tumors

Inverted papilloma

Inverted papillomas (or endophytic papillomas) are benign tumors that originate in the mucosa lining the nasal cavity and paranasal sinuses.[2] Three characteristics of inverted papillomas are (1) locally aggressive, (2) potential for carcinomatous malignant transformation, and (3) high recurrence rate.[53] On CT, they present as lobulated, isodense masses, most commonly originating in the region of the middle meatus. The site of tumor implantation can be identified by focal sclerosis of the adjacent bone, which differs from inflammatory sinonasal disease where this sclerosis is usually more diffuse. On MRI, they are isohypointense on T1-weighted images and hyperintense on T2-weighted images. The "cerebriform pattern" is a well-recognized feature on MR imaging, reported in more than 80% of cases. This refers to curvilinear polypoid folds with alternating layers of high and low signal intensity on T2-weighted and post-contrast T1-weighted images, resembling a cerebral convolution (**Fig. 12**A–C).[1,8,9]

Vascular Tumors

Juvenile nasopharyngeal angiofibroma

Juvenile nasopharyngeal angiofibroma (JNA) is a benign, slow-growing but locally aggressive vascular tumor. It occurs almost exclusively in men, commonly between

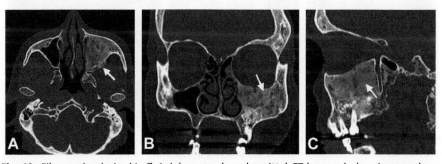

Fig. 10. Fibrous dysplasia. (*A–C*) Axial, coronal, and sagittal CT bone window images show bony obliteration and expansion of the left maxillary sinus, with the typical "ground-glass" appearance (*arrows*).

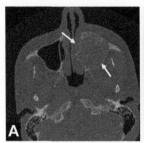
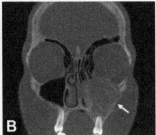
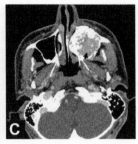

Fig. 11. Ossifying fibroma. (*A* and *B*) Axial and coronal CT bone window images show an expansile hypodense mass with foci of mineralization, involving the left maxillary sinus (*arrows*). (*C*) Axial soft-tissue window shows slight enhancement after intravenous contrast administration (*arrowhead*).

the ages of 10 and 24 years, with an average age of 15 years at diagnosis.[54,55] On CT, JNA manifests as a heterogeneous, isodense mass that is centered within the sphenopalatine foramen, with marked enhancement after intravenous contrast administration. A characteristic sign of JNA is the Holman-Miller sign, referring to anterior bowing of the posterior antral wall as the tumor fills the pterygomaxillary space.[56–58] On MRI, the lesion is hypointense on T1-weighted images and isohyperintense on T2-weighted images. On postcontrast MR images, there is marked enhancement with areas of low signal intensity that represent flow voids within the intralesional vessels (**Fig. 13**A–C).[4,9]

PRIMARY MALIGNANT NEOPLASMS
Epithelial Malignancies

Squamous cell carcinoma
SCC is the most common malignant neoplasm affecting the mucosa of the upper aerodigestive tract and represents 35% to 75% of all malignant sinonasal lesions.[9,59] It is associated with high rates of perineural spread, recurrence, and mortality.[8,12] On CT, they are seen as expansile, heterogenous, isodense lesions, with aggressive bone destruction. Advanced lesions are commonly associated with invasion of the contralateral sinonasal area, orbital wall, infratemporal fossa, and skull base. Intratumoral necrosis is also one of the characteristic findings of SCCs. On MRI, these tumors have a

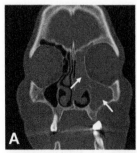
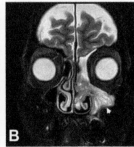
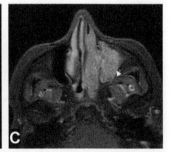

Fig. 12. Inverted papilloma. (*A*) Coronal CT bone window shows a polypoid isodense mass with increased ostium caliber and bone sclerosis at the level of ethmoid cells (*arrows*). (*B*) Coronal STIR image showing convoluted cerebriform pattern of the mass (*arrowhead*). (*C*) Axial, fat-saturated, contrast-enhanced, T1-weighted MR image demonstrating heterogeneous enhancement (*arrowhead*).

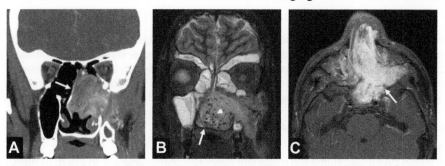

Fig. 13. JNA. (*A*) Coronal postcontrast CT soft-tissue window shows an enhancing, lobulated mass centered on the sphenopalatine foramen (*arrow*). (*B*) Coronal STIR image showing multiple flow void (*arrowhead*). (*C*) Axial, fat-saturated, contrast-enhanced, T1-weighted MR image demonstrating avid enhancement, with invasion of the sphenoid sinus and infratemporal fossa (*arrow*).

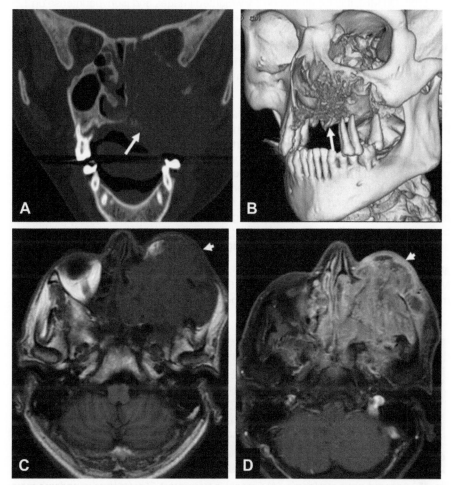

Fig. 14. SCC. (*A* and *B*) Coronal CT bone window and three-dimensional reformat showing an aggressive, expansile mass with marked infiltration of the left maxillary sinus and orbit walls (*arrow*). (*C*) Axial T1-weighted MRI showing isointense signal (*arrowhead*). (*D*) Axial, fat-saturated, contrast-enhanced, T1-weighted MRI demonstrating heterogeneous enhancement with invasive component to the skin and masticatory space (*arrowhead*).

low-to-intermediate signal intensity on T1-weighted images, a high-to-intermediate signal intensity on T2-weighted images, and heterogeneous enhancement following administration of intravenous gadolinium contrast (**Fig. 14**A–D). Up to 20% of patients present with lymph node metastasis at the time of initial presentation, mostly to the retropharyngeal nodes and levels IIA and III nodes.[1,4,7,13]

Malignant Tumors of Minor Salivary Glands

Adenoid cystic carcinoma

Adenoid cystic carcinoma is a malignant neoplasm comprising 1% to 2% of all malignant neoplasms of the head and neck. On CT, a low-grade adenoid cystic carcinoma seems as a polypoid mass that remodels surrounding bone; however, a high-grade tumor can present as a heterogeneous, expansile, destructive mass, which usually extends to the nasal cavity and occasionally to the retroantral fat, pterygopalatine fossa, and orbit. On MRI, it is isointense on T1-weighted images and isohyperintense on T2-weighted images, depending on the degree of cellularity (**Fig. 15**A–C). Adenoid cystic carcinoma is characterized by a particular propensity for perineural invasion and spread mainly through the maxillary division of the trigeminal nerve (V2). The tumor sometimes spread to intracranial components, including the cavernous sinus and trigeminal ganglion, which are located far away from the primary site.[7,8,59–61]

Adenocarcinoma

Adenocarcinomas comprise between 10% and 20% of all primary malignant tumors of the nasal cavity and paranasal sinuses. The most common location of these tumors is the ethmoidal labyrinth and the upper part of the nasal cavity (85%). On CT, they can be seen as a solid, isodense, expansile mass, occasionally exhibiting areas of calcification, reflecting the mucin content. Bone destruction is often seen in high-grade tumors. On MRI, the signal intensity of adenocarcinoma varies according to the mucin content, cellularity, and the presence of hemorrhage. Mucin-containing carcinomas are hyperintense on T2-weighted images and show gradual enhancement on contrast-enhanced T1-weighted images; however, non–mucin-containing tumors seem isohypointense on T2-weighted images (**Fig. 16**A–C).[7,8,59,62,63]

Mucoepidermoid carcinoma

Mucoepidermoid carcinoma accounts for 5% to 10% of all salivary gland tumors. The minor salivary glands located in the palatine region are the second most common site

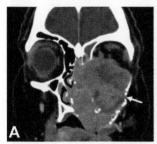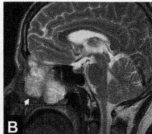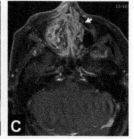

Fig. 15. Adenoid cystic carcinoma. (*A*) Coronal, postcontrast CT soft-tissue window shows a heterogeneously enhancing, expansile, sinonasal mass, with marked invasion of the orbital cavity (*arrow*). (*B*) Sagittal T2-weighted MRI sequence show hyperintense signal (*arrowhead*). (*C*) Axial, fat-saturated, contrast-enhanced, T1-weighted MRI showing heterogeneous enhancement (*arrowhead*).

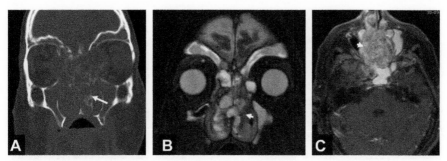

Fig. 16. Adenocarcinoma. (*A*) Coronal CT bone window shows an expansile, destructive, sinonasal mass, with opacification of the bilateral maxillary sinuses (*arrow*). (*B*) Coronal T2-weighted MR image shows heterogeneous hyperintense signal (*arrowhead*). (*C*) Axial, fat-saturated, contrast-enhanced, T1-weighted MRI demonstrating heterogenous enhancement and postobstructive secretions in the maxillary and sphenoid sinuses (*arrowhead*).

for these tumors after the parotid gland. On CT and MRI, high-grade tumors tend to seem as ill-defined, solid, expansile masses that invade the nasal cavity and pterygopalatine fossa and consequently infiltrate and destroy the hard palate region and pterygoid processes. High-grade tumors are often seen as hypoisointense lesions on T2-weighted images, indicating their high cellularity (**Fig. 17**A–C).[64–67]

Lymphoma

Non-Hodgkin lymphoma

Non-Hodgkin lymphomas (NHLs) are malignant neoplasms that account for 5% of all malignant neoplasms of the head and neck, ranking second only to SCC. Approximately 40% of NHLs may initially present with exclusive extranodal involvement. In the head and neck, primary involvement of the oral cavity is extremely rare, accounting for 2% to 5% of all extranodal lymphomas. The main affected structure of the oral cavity is the palate, with diffuse large B-cell lymphoma being the most common type (75%).[4,59]

Although NHLs are usually seen as homogeneously enhanced masses, sometimes necrotic areas are observed within the tumor, as in the case of natural killer T-cell lymphomas.[1] Bone involvement occurs in 80% of cases. On MRI, lesions are usually

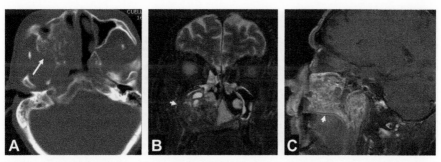

Fig. 17. Mucoepidermoid carcinoma. (*A*) Axial CT bone window shows a partially calcified, destructive mass involving the right maxillary sinus (*arrow*). (*B*) Coronal STIR image shows intermediate signal with central hyperintense cystic lesion (*arrowhead*). (*C*) Sagittal, fat-saturated, contrast-enhanced, T1-weighted MRI shows heterogenous enhancement, with involvement of the nasopharynx (*arrowhead*).

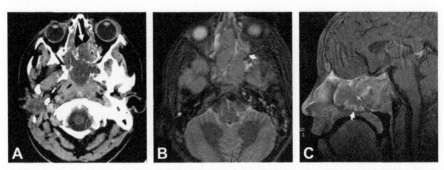

Fig. 18. Non-Hodgkin lymphoma. (*A*) Axial, postcontrast, CT soft-tissue window shows a heterogeneously enhancing, expansile mass involving the nasal and nasopharyngeal region (*arrow*). (*B*) Axial STIR image shows isointense signal (*arrowhead*). (*C*) Sagittal, fat-saturated, contrast-enhanced, T1-weighted MRI showing slight heterogenous enhancement, with involvement of the sphenoid sinus (*arrowhead*).

isointense on T1-weighted images and slightly hyperintense on T2-weighted images (**Fig. 18**A–C). Although the signal intensity is not specific, the measurement of the ADC (ADC map) helps differentiate them from other malignant tumors such as SCC.[8,9]

Sarcomas

Chondrosarcoma

Chondrosarcomas represent 0.1% of malignant neoplasms in the head and neck. The most common locations in the head and neck include the nasal cavity, maxilla, skull base, paranasal sinuses, and mandible.[8] CT findings include single or multiple hypodense areas, bony sclerosis, endostal scalloping, tumor calcifications, and enhancement after intravenous contrast. As the tumor enlarges, it invades the surrounding cortical bone and extents into adjacent soft tissues. On MRI, chondrosarcomas are isohypointense on T1-weighted images and hyperintense on T2-weighted and STIR-weighted images (**Fig. 19**A–C). Bone deposits in the tumor seem as hypointense areas on all sequences. In contrast-enhanced MRI, these tumors may enhance either uniformly or nonuniformly, depending on the amount of calcified matrix.[9,62,68]

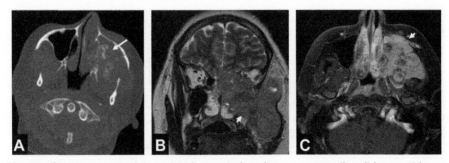

Fig. 19. Chondrosarcoma. (*A*) Axial CT bone window shows an expansile solid mass with matrix calcification (*arrow*). (*B*) Coronal T2-weighted MRI shows an isointense solid mass with intracranial, orbital, and masticatory space involvement (*arrowhead*). (*C*) Axial, fat-saturated, contrast-enhanced, T1-weighted MRI showing heterogeneous enhancement, with central hypointense areas suggestive of calcified component (*arrowhead*).

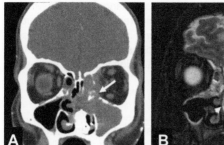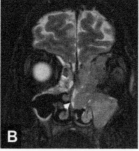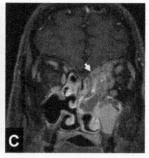

Fig. 20. Rhabdomyosarcoma. (*A*) Coronal, postcontrast CT soft-tissue window shows a mildly enhancing, infiltrative sinonasal solid mass (*arrow*). (*B*) Coronal STIR image showing intermediate signal intensity (*arrowhead*). (*C*) Coronal, fat-saturated, contrast-enhanced, T1-weighted MRI demonstrating heterogeneous enhancement, with intracranial and orbital involvement (*arrowhead*).

Rhabdomyosarcoma

Rhabdomyosarcoma is a malignant neoplasm with striated muscle differentiation. This neoplasm is one of the most common soft tissue sarcomas in neonates, children, and young adults. In children, approximately 60% of rhabdomyosarcoma cases occur in the head and neck.[8,69] On CT, rhabdomyosarcoma is seen as an isodense or slightly hypodense expansile mass, demonstrating homogeneous enhancement after intravenous contrast administration. Signs of hemorrhage and intratumoral calcifications are rarely observed. On MRI, they are isointense on T1-weighted images and moderately hyperintense on T2-weighted images (**Fig. 20**A–C). These tumors enhance variably on contrast-enhanced studies.[7,62,70,71]

Neuroectodermal Tumors

Olfactory neuroblastoma

Olfactory neuroblastoma or esthesioneuroblastoma is a neuroectodermal neoplasm originating from the olfactory epithelium in the upper nasal cavity at the level of the cribriform lamina of the ethmoid.[9,59,62] On CT, the tumor often seems as an expansile, destructive mass, containing scattered mottled calcifications. Following intravenous

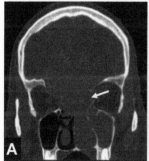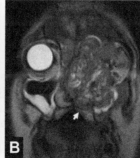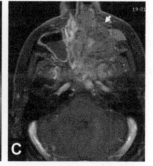

Fig. 21. Olfactory neuroblastoma. (*A*) Coronal CT bone window shows an invasive solid mass centered in cribriform plate (*arrow*). (*B*) Coronal T2-weighted MRI reveals heterogeneous signal intensity of the contents of this mass, with intracranial, maxillary, and orbital involvement (*arrowhead*). (*C*) Axial, fat-saturated, contrast-enhanced, T1-weighted MRI demonstrating heterogeneous enhancement, with deep subcutaneous tissue involvement (*arrowhead*).

contrast administration, there is diffuse and homogenous enhancement. On MRI, olfactory neuroblastoma is usually hypointense on T1-weighted images and hyperintense on T2-weighted images. On contrast MRI, there is strong homogeneous enhancement, except for occasional areas of necrosis or hemorrhage (**Fig. 21**A–C). Cystic formations at the tumor margin in its intracranial extension are highly suggestive of olfactory neuroblastoma.[4,7,8]

SUMMARY

Inflammatory polyps are the most common expansile lesions in the sinonasal cavity. CT and MRI play a complementary role in the evaluation of sinonasal pathologic condition. Imaging characteristics that are suggestive of benignity include well-defined margins, bone remodeling or sclerosis, involvement of a single paranasal sinus, homogeneity, low attenuation on CT, and high T2 signal intensity and high ADC values on MR imaging. Imaging characteristics that are suggestive of malignancy include irregular margins, erosion and bone fragmentation, extension beyond the sinus walls, high attenuation on CT, and low T2 signal intensity and low ADC values on MR imaging. Contrast-enhanced MR imaging is useful in detecting perineural tumor spread and dural invasion.

CLINICS CARE POINTS

- Imaging evaluation objective: determine whether the tumor in question is benign or malignant.
- CT and MRI play a complementary role in the evaluation of sinonasal malignant neoplasms.
- CT is highly effective in the evaluation and definition of margins and patterns of bone infiltration.
- MRI allow to distinguish the neoplasm from inflammatory changes and postobstructive secretions.
- Benign Neoplasm: well-defined margins, homogeneity, low attenuation on CT, and high T2 signal intensity and high ADC values on MR imaging.
- Malignancy: irregular margins, erosion, infiltration, high attenuation on CT, and low T2 signal intensity and low ADC values on MR imaging.

DISCLOSURE

The authors have nothing to disclose.

REFERENCES

1. Dym RJ, Masri D, Shifteh K. Imaging of the paranasal sinuses. Oral Maxillofac Surg Clin North Am 2012;24(2):175–89.
2. Whyte A, Boeddinghaus R. Imaging of adult nasal obstruction. Clin Radiol 2020; 75(9):688–704.
3. Wyler B, Mallon WK. Sinusitis update. Emerg Med Clin North Am 2019;37(1): 41–54.
4. Koeller KK. Radiologic features of sinonasal tumors. Head Neck Pathol 2016; 10(1):1–12.
5. Mahalingappa YB, Khalil HS. Sinonasal malignancy: presentation and outcomes. J Laryngol Otol 2014;128(7):654–7.

6. Jégoux F, Métreau A, Louvel G, et al. Paranasal sinus cancer. Eur Ann Otorhinolaryngol Head Neck Dis 2013;130(6):327–35.
7. Kawaguchi M, Kato H, Tomita H, et al. Imaging characteristics of malignant sinonasal tumors. J Clin Med 2017;6(12):116–31.
8. Ozturk K, Gawande R, Gencturk M, et al. Imaging features of sinonasal tumors on positron emission tomography and magnetic resonance imaging including diffusion weighted imaging: a pictorial review. Clin Imaging 2018;51:217–28.
9. Eggesbø HB. Imaging of sinonasal tumours. Cancer Imag 2012;12:136–52.
10. Rimmer J, Hellings P, Lund VJ, et al. European position paper on diagnostic tools in rhinology. Rhinology 2019;57(Suppl S28):1–41.
11. Medvedev O, Hedesiu M, Ciurea A, et al. Perineural spread in head and neck malignancies: imaging findings - an updated literature review. Bosn J Basic Med Sci 2022;22(1):22–38.
12. Bhat V, Devere J, Ramakrishanan A, et al. Perineural spread in squamous cell carcinoma of the face: an overlooked facet of information on imaging. J Maxillofac Oral Surg 2016;15(3):390–3.
13. Caillot A, Veyssière A, Ambroise B, et al. Spinal cord metastasis of squamous cell carcinoma of the maxillary sinus. Eur Ann Otorhinolaryngol Head Neck Dis 2015; 132(2):97–9.
14. Cornelius RS, Martin J, Wippold FJ 2nd, et al. ACR appropriateness criteria sinonasal disease. J Am Coll Radiol 2013;10(4):241–6.
15. Huang BY, Senior BA, Castillo M. Current trends in sinonasal imaging. Neuroimaging Clin N Am 2015;25(4):507–25.
16. Pulickal GG, Navaratnam AV, Nguyen T, et al. Imaging Sinonasal disease with MRI: providing insight over and above CT. Eur J Radiol 2018;102:157–68.
17. Das A, Bhalla AS, Sharma R, et al. Can diffusion weighted imaging aid in differentiating benign from malignant sinonasal masses? a useful adjunct. Pol J Radiol 2017;82:345–55.
18. Maheshwari N, Etikaala B, Syed AZ. Rhinolith: an incidental radiographic finding. Imaging Sci Dent 2021;51(3):333–6.
19. Seyhun N, Toprak E, Kaya KS, et al. Rhinolithiasis, a rare entity: Analysis of 31 cases and literature review. North Clin Istanb 2020;8(2):172–7.
20. Heffler E, Machetta G, Magnano M, et al. When perennial rhinitis worsens: rhinolith mimicking severe allergic rhinitis. BMJ Case Rep 2014;2014. bcr2013202539.
21. Akkoca Ö, Tüzüner A, Demirci Ş, et al. Patient characteristics and frequent localizations of rhinoliths. Turk Arch Otorhinolaryngol 2016;54(4):154–7.
22. Kose OD, Kose TE, Erdem MA, et al. Large rhinolith causing nasal obstruction. BMJ Case Rep 2015;2015. bcr2014208260.
23. Kirsch CFE, Bykowski J, Bykowski J, et al. ACR appropriateness criteria sinonasal disease. J Am Coll Radiol 2017;14(11S):S550–9.
24. Fokkens WJ, Lund VJ, Hopkins C, et al. European position paper on rhinosinusitis and nasal polyps 2020. Rhinology 2020;58(Suppl S29):1–464.
25. Joshi VM, Sansi R. Imaging in sinonasal inflammatory disease. Neuroimaging Clin N Am 2015;25(4):549–68.
26. Kastner J, Taudy M, Lisy J, et al. Orbital and intracranial complications after acute rhinosinusitis. Rhinology 2010;48(4):457–61.
27. Leo G, Triulzi F, Incorvaia C. Diagnosis of chronic rhinosinusitis. Pediatr Allergy Immunol 2012;23(Suppl 22):20–6.
28. Zojaji R, Nekooei S, Naghibi S, et al. Accuracy of limited four-slice CT-scan in diagnosis of chronic rhinosinusitis. Eur Ann Otorhinolaryngol Head Neck Dis 2015;132(6):333–5.

29. Mafee MF, Tran BH, Chapa AR. Imaging of rhinosinusitis and its complications: plain film, CT, and MRI. Clin Rev Allergy Immunol 2006;30(3):165–86.

30. Bhattacharyya N. The role of CT and MRI in the diagnosis of chronic rhinosinusitis. Curr Allergy Asthma Rep 2010;10(3):171–4.

31. Ni Mhurchu E, Ospina J, Janjua AS, et al. Fungal rhinosinusitis: a radiological review with intraoperative correlation. Can Assoc Radiol J 2017;68(2):178–86.

32. Seo YJ, Kim J, Kim K, et al. Radiologic characteristics of sinonasal fungus ball: an analysis of 119 cases. Acta Radiol 2011;52(7):790–5.

33. Newsome HA, Poetker DM. Odontogenic sinusitis: current concepts in diagnosis and treatment. Immunol Allergy Clin North Am 2020;40(2):361–9.

34. de Lima CO, Devito KL, Baraky Vasconcelos LR, et al. Correlation between endodontic infection and periodontal disease and their association with chronic sinusitis: a clinical-tomographic study. J Endod 2017;43(12):1978–83.

35. Whyte A, Boeddinghaus R. Imaging of odontogenic sinusitis. Clin Radiol 2019; 74(7):503–16.

36. Kuan EC, Suh JD. Systemic and odontogenic etiologies in chronic rhinosinusitis. Otolaryngol Clin North Am 2017;50(1):95–111.

37. Lee DH, Yoon TM, Lee JK, et al. Difference of antrochoanal polyp between children and adults. Int J Pediatr Otorhinolaryngol 2016;84:143–6.

38. Choudhury N, Hariri A, Saleh H, et al. Diagnostic challenges of antrochoanal polyps: a review of sixty-one cases. Clin Otolaryngol 2018;43(2):670–4.

39. Bidkar VG, Sajjanar AB, Patil P, et al. Role of computed tomography findings in the quest of understanding origin of antrochoanal polyp. Indian J Otolaryngol Head Neck Surg 2019;71(Suppl 3):1800–4.

40. Başer E, Sarıoğlu O, Arslan İB, et al. The effect of anatomic variations and maxillary sinus volume in antrochoanal polyp formation. Eur Arch Oto-Rhino-Laryngol 2020;277(4):1067–72.

41. Sousa DWS, Pinheiro SD, da Silva VC, et al. Bilateral antrochoanal polyps in an adult. Braz J Otorhinolaryngol 2011;77(4):539.

42. Morita S, Mizoguchi K, Iizuka K. Paranasal sinus mucoceles with visual disturbance. Auris Nasus Larynx 2010;37(6):708–12.

43. Tseng CC, Ho CY, Kao SC. Ophthalmic manifestations of paranasal sinus mucoceles. J Chin Med Assoc 2005;68(6):260–4.

44. Martel-Martín M, Gras-Cabrerizo JR, Bothe-González C, et al. Análisis clínico y resultados quirúrgicos en 58 mucoceles nasosinusales [Clinical analysis and surgical results of 58 paranasal sinus mucoceles]. Acta Otorrinolaringol Esp 2015; 66(2):92–7.

45. Dutta M. Ethmoid pneumatization and a large frontal-orbital-ethmoid mucocele. Radiology Case Reports 2019;14:419–22.

46. Alshoabi S, Gameraddin M. Giant frontal mucocele presenting with displacement of the eye globe. Radiol Case Rep 2018;13(3):627–30.

47. Bouatay R, Aouf L, Hmida B, et al. The role of imaging in the management of sinonasal mucoceles. Pan Afr Med J 2019;34:3.

48. Malard O, Gayet-Delacroix M, Jegoux F, et al. Spontaneous sphenoid sinus mucocele revealed by meningitis and brain abscess in a 12-year-old child. AJNR Am J Neuroradiol 2004;25(5):873–5.

49. Liu JJ, Thompson LD, Janisiewicz AM, et al. Ossifying fibroma of the maxilla and sinonasal tract: Case series. Allergy Rhinol (Providence) 2017;8(1):32–6.

50. Zegalie N, Speight PM, Martin L. Ossifying fibromas of the jaws and craniofacial bones. Diagn Histopathol 2015;21(9):351–8.

51. Ciniglio Appiani M, Verillaud B, Bresson D, et al. Ossifying fibromas of the paranasal sinuses: diagnosis and management. Acta Otorhinolaryngol Ital 2015; 35(5):355–61.
52. Chang HJ, Donahue JE, Sciandra KT, et al. Best cases from the AFIP: juvenile ossifying fibroma of the calvaria. Radiographics 2009;29(4):1195–9.
53. Koç N, Boyacıoğlu H, Avcu N, et al. Invasive squamous cell carcinoma arising in an inverted papilloma involving oral cavity. Oral Radiol 2020;36(2):209–14.
54. Zanation AM, Mitchell CA, Rose AS. Endoscopic skull base techniques for juvenile nasopharyngeal angiofibroma. Otolaryngol Clin North Am 2012;45(3):711–30.
55. Toplu Y, Can S, Sanlı M, et al. Middle turbinate angiofibroma: an unusual location for juvenile angiofibroma. Braz J Otorhinolaryngol 2016;84(1):122–5.
56. Mishra S, Praveena NM, Panigrahi RG, et al. Imaging in the diagnosis of juvenile nasopharyngeal angiofibroma. J Clin Imaging Sci 2013;3(Suppl 1):1.
57. Suroyo I, Budianto T. The role of diagnostic and interventional radiology in juvenile nasopharyngeal angiofibroma: a case report and literature review. Radiol Case Rep 2020;15(7):812–5.
58. Blount A, Riley KO, Woodworth BA. Juvenile nasopharyngeal angiofibroma. Otolaryngol Clin North Am 2011;44(4):989–1004.
59. Naval Baudin P, Pons Escoda A, Cos Domingo M, et al. Invasive sinonasal lesions: from the nasal fossa and paranasal sinuses to the endocranium. Curr Probl Diagn Radiol 2018;47(3):168–78.
60. Sepúlveda I, Platin E, Delgado C, et al. Sinonasal adenoid cystic carcinoma with intracranial invasion and perineural spread: a case report and review of the literature. J Clin Imaging Sci 2015;5:57.
61. Gurung S, Pathak BD, Karki S, et al. Adenoid cystic carcinoma of maxillary antrum: a case report. Int J Surg Case Rep 2022;94:107055.
62. Agarwal M, Policeni B. Sinonasal neoplasms. Semin Roentgenol 2019;54(3): 244–57.
63. Patel NN, Maina IW, Kuan EC, et al. Adenocarcinoma of the sinonasal tract: a review of the national cancer database. J Neurol Surg B Skull Base 2020;81(6): 701–8.
64. Dossani RH, Akbarian-Tefaghi H, Lemonnier L, et al. Mucoepidermoid carcinoma of palatal minor salivary glands with intracranial extension: a case report and literature review. J Neurol Surg Rep 2016;77(4):e156–9.
65. Sepúlveda I, Frelinghuysen M, Platin E, et al. Mandibular central mucoepidermoid carcinoma: a case report and review of the literature. Case Rep Oncol 2014;7(3):732–8.
66. Raut D, Khedkar S. Primary intraosseous mucoepidermoid carcinoma of the maxilla: a case report and review of literature. Dentomaxillofac Radiol 2009;38(3):163–8.
67. Hiyama T, Kuno H, Sekiya K, et al. Imaging of malignant minor salivary gland tumors of the head and neck. Radiographics 2021;41(1):175–91.
68. Wangaryattawanich P, Agarwal M, Rath T. Imaging features of cartilaginous tumors of the head and neck. J Clin Imaging Sci 2021;11:66.
69. Sepúlveda I, Spencer ML, Cabezas C, et al. Orbito-ethmoidal rhabdomyosarcoma in an adult patient: a case report and review of the literature. Case Rep Oncol 2014;7(2):513–21.
70. Zeng J, Liu L, Li J, et al. MRI features of different types of sinonasal rhabdomyosarcomas: a series of eleven cases. Dentomaxillofac Radiol 2021;50(8):20210030.
71. Zhu J, Zhang J, Tang G, et al. Computed tomography and magnetic resonance imaging observations of rhabdomyosarcoma in the head and neck. Oncol Lett 2014;8(1):155–60.

Imaging Evaluation of the Temporomandibular Joint

Galal Omami, BDS, MSc, MDentSc, FRCD(C), Dip. ABOMR[a],*,
Craig S. Miller, DMD, MS[b]

KEYWORDS

- Temporomandibular joint • Diagnostic imaging • Computed tomography • MRI

KEY POINTS

- Interpreting temporomandibular joint (TMJ) imaging studies requires an understanding of both the anatomy and pathophysiology of the joint and surrounding structures.
- Panoramic radiography remains the most useful screening tool for TMJ dysfunction.
- CT and MR imaging are often complementary in the evaluation of the TMJ.
- Contrast medium administration in MR imaging is essential to assess the existence of active synovitis.
- Skeletal scintigraphy has been shown as a useful modality for assessing the bone activity in condylar hyperplasia.

INTRODUCTION

The temporomandibular joint (TMJ) is a complex joint composed of the head of mandibular condyle and the glenoid fossa and articular eminence of the temporal bone. The joint space is separated into superior and inferior spaces or compartments by a dense fibrous disc (meniscus) interposed between the condylar and temporal components. The articulating surfaces of both bones are covered with a thin layer of fibrocartilage. The joint is encased by a fibrous capsule, which is lined by synovial membrane. In the sagittal plane, the disc has a biconcave "bow tie" shape with thick anterior and posterior bands and a thin central part. The periphery of the disc is attached to the inner surface of the joint capsule. The anterior band merges with the superior head of the lateral pterygoid muscle. The posterior band is attached to the condyle and to the temporal bone by the posterior disc attachment. This attachment is also referred to as the retrodiscal tissues or bilaminar zone, and it contains neurovascular structures. In the closed-mouth position, the disc is positioned with the posterior thick band immediately superior to

[a] Division of Oral Diagnosis, Oral Medicine, and Oral Radiology, Department of Oral Health Practice, University of Kentucky College of Dentistry, 770 Rose Street, D-140, Lexington, KY 40536, USA; [b] Division of Oral Diagnosis, Oral Medicine, and Oral Radiology, University of Kentucky College of Dentistry, 770 Rose Street, D-140, Lexington, KY 40536, USA
* Corresponding author.
E-mail address: galal.omami@uky.edu

Dent Clin N Am 68 (2024) 357–373
https://doi.org/10.1016/j.cden.2023.10.001
0011-8532/24/© 2023 Elsevier Inc. All rights reserved.

dental.theclinics.com

the condyle and the thin central part between the anterosuperior surface of the condyle and the posterior surface of the articular eminence. In the open-mouth position, the central part of the disc sits between the condyle and articular eminence (**Fig.** 1A and B). Mandibular opening involves rotation and forward translation (sliding) of the condyle. Rotation and translation occur in the superior and inferior joint spaces. However, rotation occurs predominantly in the inferior joint space, and translation is more evident in the superior joint space.

Disorders of the TMJ include developmental and acquired abnormalities that result in altered morphology or function of the joint (**Box 1**). Imaging is an important adjunct to the clinical examination and is particularly valuable in the diagnosis of TMJ disorders.

Panoramic radiography is recommended for initial imaging assessment of the osseous structures of the TMJ and may suggest the need for further radiologic examinations such as cone-beam computed tomography (CBCT) or multidetector computed tomography (MDCT). In a normal TMJ, the articulating surfaces appear smoothly curved, with thick and regular cortication. MRI may be performed for visualizing the disc and other soft tissues of the joint.[1,2] This article describes the various abnormalities that affect the osseous and soft tissue structures of the TMJ and covers internal derangement, arthritides, and developmental abnormalities, as well as tumors and tumor-like conditions.

Internal Derangement

Definition and clinical features

Internal derangement is a nonspecific term referring to an abnormality in the soft tissue components of the joint resulting in altered function, which typically includes disc displacement. A displaced disc may become deformed or be associated with other signs of TMJ dysfunction such as adhesion and effusion. The cause of internal derangement is unknown, but parafunctional habits, mandibular trauma, and whiplash injury have been implicated as predisposing factors. The disc most often displaces in an anterior direction. Thus, when the teeth are in the closed-mouth position, the

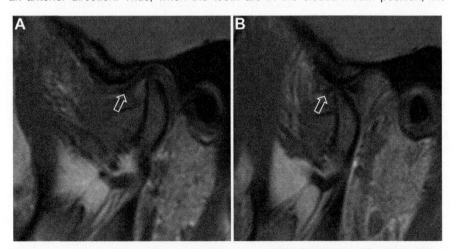

Fig. 1. Normal disc mobility. (*A*) Sagittal oblique T1-weighted MR image (closed-mouth position) shows a disc (*arrow*) in its normal position between the condyle and temporal bone. (*B*) Sagittal oblique T1-weighted MR image shows the disc (*arrow*) has maintained its normal position at the open-mouth position.

Box 1
Disorders of the temporomandibular joint

Internal derangement
  Disc displacement
  Disc deformity

Developmental abnormalities
  Condylar hyperplasia
  Condylar hypoplasia
  Bifid condyle

Arthritic conditions
  Degenerative joint disease
  Rheumatoid arthritis
  Juvenile idiopathic arthritis
  Septic arthritis
  Psoriatic arthritis

Tumor-like conditions
  Synovial chondromatosis
  Chondrocalcinosis
  Pigmented villonodular synovitis

Hypermobility
  Subluxation
  Dislocation

Hypomobility
  Adhesion
  Ankylosis

Trauma
  Hemarthrosis
  Fractures

Tumors
  Benign
  Malignant

posterior band of the disc is positioned in front of the condyle, instead of sitting in position directly superior to the condyle. When an anteriorly displaced disc reverts to its normal position at maximum mouth opening, this condition is known as anterior disc displacement with reduction and is usually associated with reciprocal clicking noises (**Fig. 2**A and B). If the disc remains anteriorly displaced on opening, it is diagnosed as anterior disc displacement without reduction (**Fig. 3**A and B). In the early stage, this condition is associated with limitation of mandibular opening (closed lock) and deviation of the mandible to the affected side on opening. With time, the opening capacity of the TMJ improves as a result of stretching of the posterior disc attachment.

Imaging features
The standard MR imaging protocol for the TMJ includes oblique sagittal and oblique coronal images perpendicular and parallel to the long axis of the condylar head, respectively. Sagittal images are acquired in both closed- and open-mouth positions to determine the mobility of the disc. Coronal images are obtained only in the closed-mouth position to determine mediolateral displacement of the disc. The examinations usually are performed with the use of T1-weighted, proton-density-weighted, and T2-weighted sequences.[1] Proton-density images are superior to T1-weighted images in demonstrating the disc relative to the surrounding cortical bone. T2-weighted images

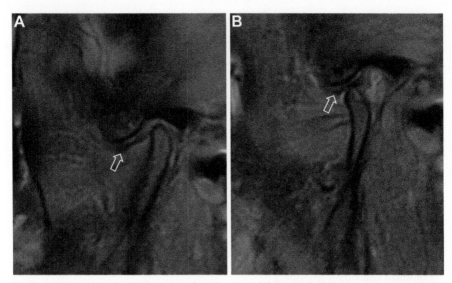

Fig. 2. Anterior disc displacement with reduction. (*A*) Sagittal oblique proton-density MR image (closed-mouth position) shows an anteriorly displaced disc (*arrow*). (*B*) Sagittal oblique proton-density MR image (open-mouth position) shows the disc (*arrow*) has returned to its normal position between the condyle and articular eminence.

are valuable in identifying joint effusion and inflammatory changes in the joint capsule. Although contrast-enhanced MR imaging is usually not indicated for the evaluation of disc abnormalities, it can be useful in differentiating active synovitis from joint effusion.[3]

Other Findings Related to Internal Derangement

Joint effusion
Effusion is an abnormal accumulation of synovial fluid within the joint and may be associated with disc displacement or arthritic conditions. The presence of joint

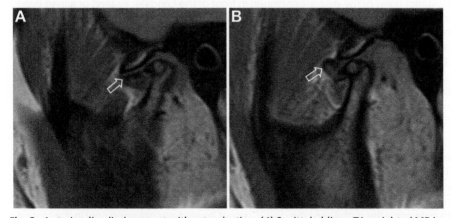

Fig. 3. Anterior disc displacement without reduction. (*A*) Sagittal oblique T1-weighted MR image (closed-mouth position) shows the disc (*arrow*) anterior to the condyle. (*B*) Sagittal oblique T1-weighted MR image (open-mouth position) shows the disc (*arrow*) remaining anterior to the condyle. The disc is folding against the joint capsule. The condyle shows degenerative changes manifesting as flattening, osteophyte formation "beaking," and subchondral erosion.

effusion is a usual finding in symptomatic individuals. Effusion is best seen on T2-weighted MR images (**Fig. 4**). These images also may be useful for highlighting disc perforation because of the arthrographic effect created by the high signal intensity of the fluid.[3]

Intra-articular adhesions
Fibrous adhesions in the TMJ may develop in advanced cases of internal derangement. Adhesions may restrict movement of the disc relative to the temporal joint component (ie, stuck disc), resulting in a closed lock.[4] MRI does not directly identify the adhesions, but the fixed disc position is suggestive. Arthroscopy is a minimally invasive surgical technique that allows for both direct visualization and treatment of intra-articular adhesions (**Fig. 5**).[5]

Condylar Hyperplasia

Definition and clinical features
Condylar hyperplasia is a developmental abnormality characterized by asymmetric overgrowth of the mandibular condyle. The cause is uncertain, although several etiologic factors have been suggested, including trauma, infection, hormonal disturbances, hypervascularity, and heredity.[2,6] Condylar hyperplasia is noted most frequently in adolescents and young adults, with a female predominance. The condition is usually associated with varying degrees of ipsilateral mandibular hyperplasia. The clinical examination may reveal facial asymmetry and deviation of the mandible to the unaffected side. As a result, patients may have a posterior open bite on the affected side or a crossbite on the unaffected side. The maxilla on the affected side may grow downward to meet the mandible, resulting in an occlusal cant downward on the affected side.[6]

Imaging features
Radiographically, the affected condyle may be normal in shape and structure but is increased in size, and the glenoid fossa is proportionally large (**Fig. 6**). The condylar neck may be elongated and thickened. Compensatory changes such as lateral

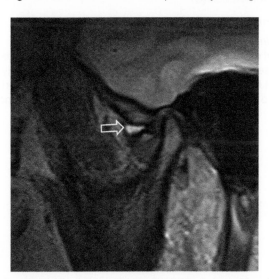

Fig. 4. Joint effusion. Sagittal oblique T2-weighted MR image (closed-mouth position) shows high signal intensity fluid in the upper joint space (*arrow*).

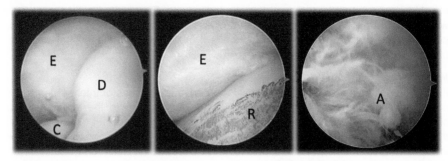

Fig. 5. Arthroscopic views of the TMJ. A, adhesions; C, condylar head; D, disc; E, eminence; R, retrodiscal tissue. (*Courtesy of* Melvyn Yeoh, MD, DMD, Lexington, KY).

bending of the elongated condylar neck and downward bowing of the inferior mandibular border often occur.[2] Secondary bone remodeling or degenerative changes may be seen in the affected joint. Bone scintigraphy may be helpful in assessing growth activity in condylar hyperplasia (**Fig. 7**).[6]

Bifid Condyle

Definition and clinical features
Bifid condyle is a rare developmental anomaly characterized by a double-headed mandibular condyle. The cause of this condition is unknown, although trauma has been suggested as playing an etiologic role.[7] The orientation of the bifid condyle may be mediolateral or anteroposterior. The condition is typically asymptomatic and is more often unilateral.

Imaging features
Radiographic examination will demonstrate a bilobed appearance of the condylar head (**Fig. 8**). The glenoid fossa may be remodeled (enlarged) in response to the abnormal condylar morphology.

Degenerative Joint Disease

Definition and clinical features
Degenerative joint disease (DJD), also known as osteoarthritis or osteoarthrosis, is the most common disease affecting the TMJ. It represents approximately 11% of patients evaluated for TMJ pain.[8] The pathologic process is characterized by progressive degradation of the articular cartilage and remodeling of the subchondral bone. These

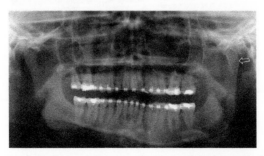

Fig. 6. Condylar hyperplasia. Panoramic image shows condylar hyperplasia involving the left condyle (*arrow*). Note the secondary hyperplasia of the same side of the mandible.

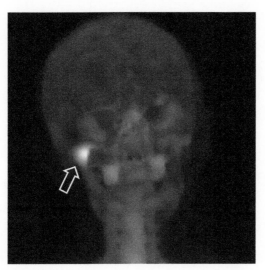

Fig. 7. Condylar hyperplasia. Technetium bone scan demonstrates increased bone activity in the right condyle (*arrow*).

changes are believed to result from abnormal remodeling due to decreased adaptive capability of the joint and/or functional loading of the joint that exceeds the normal adaptive capability. However, it is now generally accepted that there is an inflammatory component to the disease.[9] DJD may be associated with many etiologic factors, including trauma, parafunction, unstable occlusion, and increased joint friction. Disc displacement may also be a contributing factor.[10] The incidence of DJD increases with age and shows a female predominance. Patients may be asymptomatic, or they may have signs and symptoms of TMJ dysfunction, including pain, tenderness, crepitus, limited range of motion, and muscle pain.

Imaging features
DJD is characterized radiographically by flattening and erosion of the articulating surfaces, osteophyte (spur) formation, subchondral cyst-like erosion (Ely cyst), subchondral sclerosis, and loss of joint space (**Fig. 9**). Osteophyte formation occurs at the periphery of the articulating surfaces, most often on the anterior aspect of the condyle. Osteophytes may break off and become loose bodies within the joint.

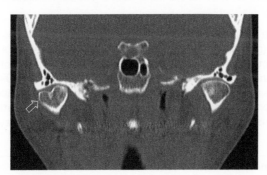

Fig. 8. Bifid condyle. Coronal CT image shows a notch in the superior condylar surface, giving a heart-shaped condyle (*arrow*).

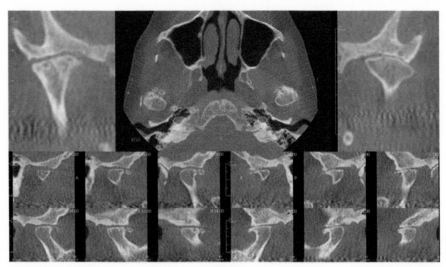

Fig. 9. Degenerative joint disease. Standard TMJ reformatted display incorporating coronal, axial reference, and serial cross-sectional images show prominent osteophyte formation at the anterior aspect of the condyles, flattening, subchondral sclerosis, and erosions of all articulating surfaces, with diminished width of the joint space.

Juvenile Idiopathic Arthritis

Definition and clinical features

Juvenile idiopathic arthritis (JIA), formerly known as juvenile rheumatoid arthritis or juvenile chronic arthritis, is a chronic rheumatologic inflammatory disease that manifests before age 16 years.[11] It results in inflammation of the synovium and destruction of the hard and soft tissues of the joints. JIA occurs more frequently in women. Single or multiple joints can be affected. Unilateral or bilateral TMJ involvement occurs in about 50% of patients diagnosed with JIA.[12] Signs and symptoms include pain, tenderness, swelling, morning stiffness, and decreased range of jaw motion. Severe involvement of both TMJs results in inhibited mandibular growth. Affected patients may have retrognathia, posteroinferior rotation of the mandible, loss of posterior facial height, anterior open bite malocclusion, and convex facial profile.[6] Unilateral TMJ involvement may result in facial asymmetry and deviation of the mandible to the affected side. Patients may be seronegative for rheumatoid factor and antinuclear antibodies.[11]

Imaging features

MR imaging is the optimal modality for the diagnosis of JIA. The use of intravenous contrast medium (gadolinium) is essential to assess the existence of active synovitis (**Fig. 10**).[11] Characteristic MRI findings include synovial enhancement and thickening, joint effusion, bone marrow edema, and disc abnormalities.[13] Osseous changes consist of progressive erosions of the condyle and articular eminence. The condyles may have an abnormal anterior position because of erosion of the articular eminence. Fibrous or bony fusion of opposing articular surfaces (ankylosis) may occur.

Septic Arthritis

Definition and clinical features

Infection of the TMJ is rare and is thought to result from the spread of disease from another region to the joint by direct or hematogenous route. Infection may also arise

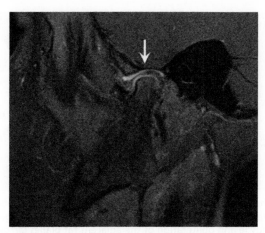

Fig. 10. Juvenile idiopathic arthritis. Sagittal contrast-enhanced T1-weighted MR image shows enhancement due to synovitis (*arrow*). (*From* Aiken A, Bouloux G, Hudgins P. MR imaging of the temporomandibular joint. Magn Reson Imaging Clin N Am. 2012 Aug;20(3):397 to 412; with permission).

after trauma or surgery to the TMJ.[14] Septic arthritis usually occurs unilaterally. Patients complain of pain and swelling over the affected joint, trismus, cervical lymphadenopathy, fever, and malaise. Depending on the severity of infection, varying degrees of joint destruction may occur. Later in the disease, joint fibrosis and ankylosis may develop.[15] In children, the disease may affect the growth potential of the condyle, resulting in mandibular asymmetry and malocclusion.

Imaging features
No radiographic changes may be present in acute stages of the disease, although the joint space may be widened as a result of joint effusion. The initial changes of septic arthritis may include rarefaction of the condyle and temporal component. With time, the bone rarefaction becomes more profound, sequestra may be present, and there may be sclerosis and periosteal reaction.[2] Contrast-enhanced CT may show associated inflammatory changes, such as increased attenuation of periarticular fat, loss of fat planes, abscess formation, and enlargement of surrounding muscles (**Fig. 11**A and B). MR imaging may demonstrate joint effusion, synovial enhancement and thickening, and bone marrow edema.

Synovial Chondromatosis

Definition and clinical features
Synovial chondromatosis is an uncommon nonneoplastic condition characterized by metaplastic formation of cartilaginous nodules within the synovial membrane of joints. These nodules may enlarge and eventually detach to become loose intra-articular bodies.[16] The intra-articular bodies often become calcified and may ossify. When this occurs, the term synovial osteochondromatosis may be used. The condition is most common in middle-aged adults and demonstrates a female predilection. Although most cases are unilateral, bilateral involvement may occur.[17] Patients frequently complain of pain, periarticular swelling, and limitation of joint motion.

Imaging features
Radiographic findings include multiple intra-articular calcified loose bodies of similar size and shape, widening of the joint space, and erosive and sclerotic changes in

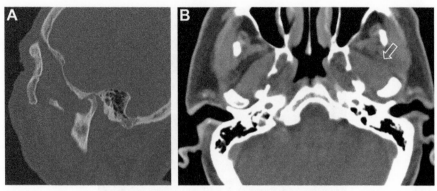

Fig. 11. Septic arthritis. (*A*) Sagittal CT bone window image shows lytic changes of the mandibular condyle. (*B*) Axial soft-tissue window image shows enlargement of the left lateral pterygoid muscle and obliteration of the adjacent fat planes (*arrow*). These findings are consistent with an inflammatory process. (*Courtesy of* Richard Wiggins, MD, Salt Lake City, UT).

the condyle and glenoid fossa (**Fig. 12**A–C). The individual bodies may have a peripheral cortex and radiolucent core reflecting their bony nature. CT is the optimal imaging modality to identify and characterize these calcified fragments and erosion and sclerosis of bone.[18] Intra-articular calcifications, however, are not specific and may be seen in other disorders, such as DJD, chondrocalcinosis, osteochondritis dissecans, and chondrosarcoma.[2,16] The absence of intra-articular calcifications does not preclude a diagnosis of synovial chondromatosis. Expansion of the articular capsule and joint effusion are common findings in patients with synovial chondromatosis, and these findings can best be demonstrated on MR imaging.[16]

Chondrocalcinosis

Definition and clinical features

Chondrocalcinosis, which is also known as calcium pyrophosphate deposition disease or pseudogout, is a rare benign arthropathy characterized by precipitation of calcium pyrophosphate dihydrate crystals in articular and periarticular tissues. Several metabolic conditions are identified as risk factors for chondrocalcinosis. These include hyperparathyroidism, hypophosphatasia, hemochromatosis, and hypomagnesemia.[19] TMJ involvement is usually unilateral, but occasionally both sides may be affected. Most cases have been reported in middle-aged and older adults.[20] Patients may experience pain and swelling over the TMJ area with limitation of mouth opening.

Imaging features

Chondrocalcinosis appears on images as fine calcifications within the joint space (**Fig. 13**). The osseous components of the joint may exhibit a mixture of bone sclerosis and erosion. More severe cases can present with significant erosion of the glenoid fossa. CT is the best method for demonstrating the intra-articular calcifications and assessing the severity of the disease.[1] The utility of MR imaging in the diagnosis of chondrocalcinosis is limited.

Pigmented Villonodular Synovitis

Definition and clinical features

Pigmented villonodular synovitis is a rare, benign, yet potentially locally aggressive disease or tumor characterized by synovial proliferation and hemarthrosis. The condition

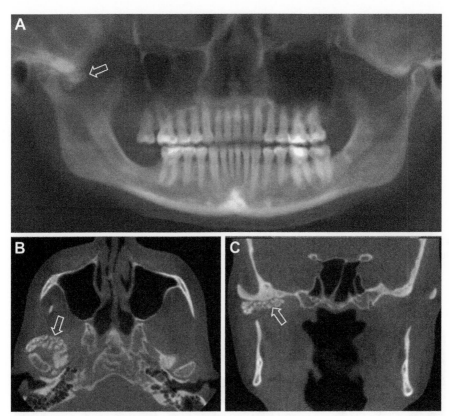

Fig. 12. Synovial osteochondromatosis. Reformated panoramic (*A*), axial (*B*), and coronal (*C*) cone-beam CT images show innumerable ossified bodies, of similar size and shape, surrounding the right condylar head (*arrows*). (Images are courtesy of Dr. Marcel Noujeim, DDS, MS, Oral and maxillofacial Radiologist, San Antonio, Texas, USA.)

usually arises in the third and fourth decades without a significant sex predilection. In most instances, it is monoarticular, although it may affect more than one joint.[21] Pain and swelling are common features.

Imaging features
On CT, the lesion usually presents as a hyperdense mass, which in turn can cause bone erosion on both sides of the TMJ.[22] The enlarging mass may erode through the contiguous skull base to extend intracranially. MR imaging demonstrates low signal intensity on T1-, T2-, and proton-density-weighted sequences because of hemosiderin deposition (**Fig. 14**A–C). The magnetic susceptibility artifact from hemosiderin in these lesions as seen on T2* sequences is virtually pathognomonic.[23]

Dislocation

Definition and clinical features
Dislocation of the TMJ is a nonreducing displacement of the condyle outside its functional limits within the glenoid fossa and posterior slope of the articular eminence. It usually occurs bilaterally and in an anterior direction. Dislocation can occur as a result of trauma or iatrogenic factors, such as a lengthy dental procedure or endotracheal

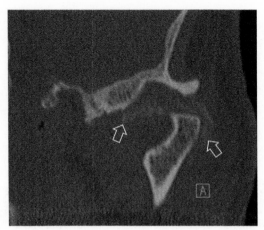

Fig. 13. Chondrocalcinosis. Coronal bone-window CT image shows faintly calcified material surrounding the condylar head (*arrows*). (*Courtesy* of Richard Wiggins, MD, Salt Lake City, UT.)

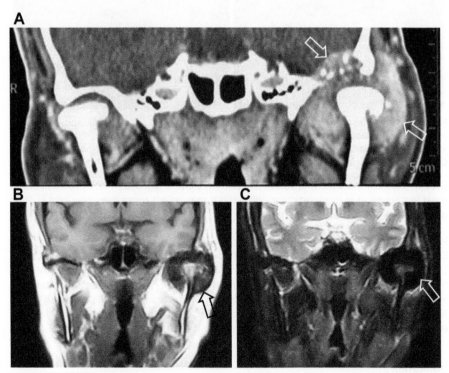

Fig. 14. Pigmented villonodular synovitis. (*A*) Coronal post-contrast CT image shows an enhancing mass in the left TMJ. The mass is extending from the joint and eroding through the glenoid fossa (*arrows*). T1-weighted (*B*) and T2-weighted (*C*) MR images show low signal intensity (*arrows*) representing hemosiderin deposition. (*From* Cai J, Cai Z, Gao Y. Pigmented villonodular synovitis of the temporomandibular joint: a case report and the literature review. Int J Oral Maxillofac Surg. 2011;40(11):1314 to 22; with permission.)

intubation.[24] Patients are unable to close the mouth. Acute dislocation is often associated with severe muscle spasm and pain.

Imaging features

Panoramic and CT images (either CBCT or MDCT) are useful for evaluation of TMJ dislocation. Diagnostic images show the condyle positioned anterior and superior to the articular eminence (**Fig. 15A–C**).

Ankylosis

Definition and clinical features

Ankylosis is a condition in which condylar movement is restricted because of fibrous or bony fusion of the opposing surfaces of the joint. Most cases are caused by trauma, infection, radiotherapy, or severe arthritic condition. Ankylosis results in a gradually worsening inability to open the mouth, with the mandible deviating toward the affected

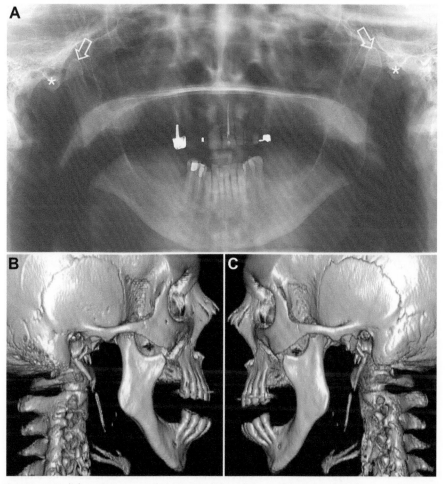

Fig. 15. TMJ dislocation. Panoramic image (*A*) and three-dimensional surface rendering CT image in lateral orientation (*B, C*) demonstrate bilateral condylar dislocation (open lock). Both condyles (*arrows*) are positioned outside the glenoid fossae, anterior and superior to the articular eminences (*asterisks*).

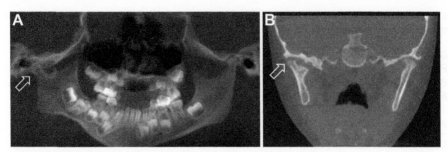

Fig. 16. Fibrous ankylosis. Reformatted panoramic (*A*) and coronal (*B*) cone-beam CT images show deformity of the right TMJ (*arrows*). Note the irregular articulating surfaces of the condyle and glenoid fossa with maintenance of the joint space, suggesting fibrous ankylosis. There is an associated mandibular hypoplasia with a decreased vertical height of the ramus and deepened antegonial notch on the affected side.

side on opening. Children who develop ankylosis may have facial asymmetry because of diminished mandibular growth on the affected side (**Fig. 16**A and B).[6] Pain is not a common feature in ankylosis. Extra-articular causes of restricted mouth opening include muscle spasm or fibrosis, myositis ossificans, and hyperplasia or a tumor of the coronoid process (**Fig. 17**).[2]

Imaging features

CT is preferred over MR imaging for demonstration of TMJ ankylosis. In fibrous ankylosis, the opposing articulating surfaces are usually irregular and appear to fit one another in a jigsaw puzzle fashion. In bony ankylosis, the joint space may be partially

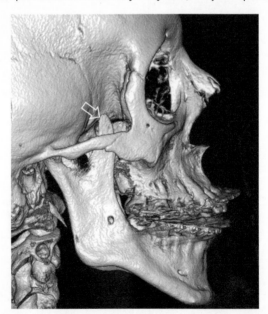

Fig. 17. Coronoid hyperplasia. Three-dimensional reconstructed cone-beam CT scan in lateral orientation shows elongation of the coronoid process (*arrow*), with its tip extending above the superior rim of the zygomatic arch. (*A*) hyperplastic coronoid process impinging on the inner surface of zygoma can cause limitation of opening, and the diagnosis can be confirmed by performing the scan in the open-mouth position.

or completely obliterated by osseous material. Usually, there is compensatory hyper-plasia of the coronoid processes.[25]

Osteochondroma

Definition and clinical features
Osteochondroma is one of the most common benign tumors of the TMJ. It consists of a sessile or pedunculated bony outgrowth with a cartilaginous cap. The cortical and med-ullary components of the osteochondroma are continuous with those of the underlaying native bone.[26] The mean age at diagnosis is 40 years. Women are affected more frequently than men. Patients with condylar osteochondroma may have facial asymme-try, TMJ dysfunction, and malocclusion.[27] Osteochondroma of the coronoid process may impinge on the zygomatic bone, resulting in limited mandibular opening.[28]

Imaging features
Osteochondroma usually appears as a nodular or mushroom-shaped bony mass (**Fig. 18**). Occasionally, a condylar osteochondroma may give the appearance of a hy-perplastic condyle, but with irregular cortical outline and abnormal internal structure. The cartilaginous cap is not seen on plain films or CT. The tumor has a heterogenous low to intermediate signal intensity on T1- and T2-weighted MR images.[26]

Malignant Tumors

Definition and clinical features
Malignant tumors of the TMJs may be primary or secondary. Primary malignant tu-mors of the TMJ are exceedingly rare and include osteosarcoma, chondrosarcoma, fibrosarcoma, and synovial sarcoma. Secondary malignant tumors may involve the TMJ either via direct invasion from an adjacent primary neoplasm or hematogenous metastasis from distant primary tumors. The most common metastatic lesions include carcinomas arising in the breast, lung, kidney, colon, and prostate.[29] Patients with ma-lignant tumors (either primary or metastatic) may be asymptomatic, or they may complain of signs and symptoms of TMJ dysfunction.

Imaging features
Primary and metastatic malignant tumors manifest as a destructive process with or without induction of bone formation (**Fig. 19**A and B). Chondrosarcoma may show bone destruction with a rim of faint calcifications, often simulating the appearance of the articular loose bodies that occurs in chondrocalcinosis.[2] Some tumors, such as osteosarcoma and prostate and breast metastatic lesions, can stimulate a

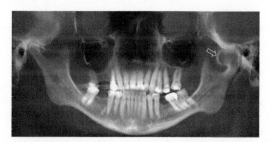

Fig. 18. Condylar osteochondroma. Reconstructed panoramic image from cone-beam CT volume shows an osteochondroma involving the left condylar head (*arrow*). Note the cortical and internal aspects of the osteochondroma are continuous with those of the condylar head.

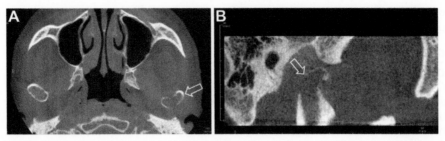

Fig. 19. Metastatic carcinoma. Axial (*A*) and sagittal (*B*) cone-beam CT images show ill-defined bone destruction of the left condyle (*arrows*) related to a metastatic colon carcinoma.

periosteal reaction that usually takes the form of a spiculated pattern. CT and MRI usually demonstrate a soft-tissue mass that enhances with intravenous contrast and frequently associated with bone destruction.

SUMMARY

Interpreting TMJ imaging studies requires an understanding of both the anatomy and pathophysiology of the joint and surrounding structures. Panoramic radiography remains the most useful screening tool for TMJ dysfunction. CT and MR imaging are often complementary in the evaluation of the TMJ. Osseous changes are more precisely studied with CT. Disc abnormalities, joint effusions, and inflammatory changes of the capsule are best evaluated with MRI. Contrast medium administration in MR imaging is essential to assess the existence of active synovitis. Skeletal scintigraphy has been shown as a useful modality for assessing the bone activity in condylar hyperplasia but not particularly helpful for diagnosis of TMJ disorders.

DISCLOSURE

The authors declare that they have no conflict of interest.

REFERENCES

1. Westesson PL, Otonari-Yamamoto M, Sano T, et al. Anatomy, pathology, and imaging of the temporomandibular joint. In: Som PM, Curtin HD, editors. Head and neck imaging. 5th edition. St. Louis, MO: Mosby; 2011. p. 1547–613.
2. Perschbacher S. Temporomandibular joint abnormalities. In: White S, Pharoah M, editors. Oral radiology: principles and interpretation. 7th edition. St Louis (MO): Elsevier; 2014. p. 492–523.
3. Tomas X, Pomes J, Berenguer J, et al. MR imaging of temporomandibular joint dysfunction: a pictorial review. Radiographics 2006;26(3):765–81.
4. Rao VM, Liem MD, Farole A, et al. Elusive "stuck" disk in the temporomandibular joint: diagnosis with MR imaging. Radiology 1993;189(3):823–7.
5. McCain JP, Hossameldin RH. Advanced arthroscopy of the temporomandibular joint. Atlas Oral Maxillofac Surg Clin North Am 2011;19(2):145–67.
6. Chouinard AF, Kaban LB, Peacock ZS. Acquired Abnormalities of the Temporomandibular Joint. Oral Maxillofac Surg Clin North Am 2018;30(1):83–96.
7. Antoniades K, Hadjipetrou L, Antoniades V, et al. Bilateral bifid mandibular condyle. Oral Surg Oral Med Oral Pathol Oral Radiol Endod 2004;97(4):535–8.
8. Tanaka E, Detamore MS, Mercuri LG. Degenerative disorders of the temporomandibular joint: etiology, diagnosis, and treatment. J Dent Res 2008;87(4):296–307.

9. Wang XD, Zhang JN, Gan YH, et al. Current understanding of pathogenesis and treatment of TMJ osteoarthritis. J Dent Res 2015;94(5):666–73.
10. Larheim TA, Hol C, Ottersen MK, et al. The Role of imaging in the diagnosis of temporomandibular joint pathology. Oral Maxillofac Surg Clin North Am 2018; 30(3):239–49.
11. Navallas M, Inarejos EJ, Iglesias E, et al. MR imaging of the temporomandibular joint in juvenile idiopathic arthritis: technique and findings. Radiographics 2017; 37(2):595–612.
12. Stoll ML, Sharpe T, Beukelman T, et al. Risk factors for temporomandibular joint arthritis in children with juvenile idiopathic arthritis. J Rheumatol 2012;39:1880–7.
13. Abramowicz S, Cheon JE, Kim S, et al. Magnetic resonance imaging of temporo-mandibular joints in children with arthritis. J Oral Maxillofac Surg 2011;69(9): 2321–8.
14. Omiunu A, Talmor G, Nguyen B, et al. Septic arthritis of the temporomandibular joint: a systematic review. J Oral Maxillofac Surg 2021;79(6):1214–29.
15. Gayle EA, Young SM, McKenna SJ, et al. Septic arthritis of the temporomandib-ular joint: case reports and review of the literature. J Emerg Med 2013;45:674–8.
16. Herzog S, Mafee M. Synovial chondromatosis of the TMJ: MR and CT findings. AJNR Am J Neuroradiol 1990;11(4):742–5.
17. Guijarro-Martínez R, Puche Torres M, Marqués Mateo M, et al. Bilateral synovial chondromatosis of the temporomandibular joint. J Cranio-Maxillo-Fac Surg 2011;39(4):261–5.
18. Murphey MD, Vidal JA, Fanburg-Smith JC, et al. Imaging of synovial chondroma-tosis with radiologic-pathologic correlation. Radiographics 2007;27(5):1465–88.
19. Rosenthal AK, Ryan LM. Calcium pyrophosphate deposition disease. N Engl J Med 2016;374(26):2575–84.
20. Willekens I, Fares A, Devos H, et al. Prevalence of chondrocalcinosis in the temporomandibular joint in patients with chondrocalcinosis of the knee or wrist. Dentomaxillofac Radiol 2020;49(7):20190450.
21. Masih S, Antebi A. Imaging of pigmented villonodular synovitis. Semin Musculos-kelet Radiol 2003;7(3):205–16.
22. Le WJ, Li MH, Yu Q, et al. Pigmented villonodular synovitis of the temporomandib-ular joint: CT imaging findings. Clin Imaging 2014;38(1):6–10.
23. Kim KW, Han MH, Park SW, et al. Pigmented villonodular synovitis of the tempo-romandibular joint: MR findings in four cases. Eur J Radiol 2004;49(3):229–34.
24. Liddell A, Perez DE. Temporomandibular joint dislocation. Oral Maxillofac Surg Clin North Am 2015;27(1):125–36.
25. Wang WH, Xu B, Zhang BJ, et al. Temporomandibular joint ankylosis contributing to coronoid process hyperplasia. Int J Oral Maxillofac Surg 2016;45(10):1229–33.
26. Murphey MD, Choi JJ, Kransdorf MJ, et al. Imaging of osteochondroma: variants and complications with radiologic-pathologic correlation. Radiographics 2000; 20(5):1407–34.
27. Meng Q, Chen S, Long X, et al. The clinical and radiographic characteristics of condylar osteochondroma. Oral Surg Oral Med Oral Pathol Oral Radiol 2012; 114(1):e66–74.
28. Etöz OA, Alkan A, Yikilmaz A. Osteochondroma of the mandibular coronoid pro-cess: a rare cause of limited mouth opening. Br J Oral Maxillofac Surg 2009; 47(5):409–11.
29. Hirshberg A, Leibovich P, Buchner A. Metastatic tumors to the jawbones: analysis of 390 cases. J Oral Pathol Med 1994;23(8):337–41.

Soft Tissue Calcifications in the Head and Neck Region

Ali Z. Syed, BDS, MHA, MS*

KEYWORDS

- Calcification • Cone-beam computed tomography • Head • Neck • Soft tissue
- Diagnostic imaging • Calcium metabolsim disorder
- Monckeberg medial calcific sclerosis

KEY POINTS

- Because of its higher spatial resolution, Cone Beam Computed Tomography (CBCT) is more effective than conventional 2D imaging in detecting soft tissue calcifications.
- Dental practitioners should be able to differentiate the different calcifications observed on dental imaging.
- Although most soft tissue calcifications are likely incidental findings on imaging studies, some can occasionally be serious conditions that may require a physician referral or surgical intervention.

INTRODUCTION

Clinicians frequently encounter soft tissue calcifications (STCs) in their day-to-day practices. These STCs are classified into dystrophic, iatrogenic, metastatic, and idiopathic. Most STCs are asymptomatic and discovered as incidental findings on radiographic images.

This article provides an overview of STCs in the head and neck region as noted on dental imaging, with particular focus on the radiographic appearance of these entities. For simplicity, STCs are organized by region as follows: the cranial cavity, facial skin, nasopharynx, maxillary sinus, nasal region, perimandibular region, and neck region.

Cranial Cavity

STCs in the cranial cavity encompass a spectrum of radiological findings with diverse underlying etiologic factors.

Oral and Maxillofacial Medicine and Diagnostic Sciences, School of Dental Medicine - Case Western Reserve University, 9601 Chester Avenue, Cleveland, OH 44106, USA
* Corresponding author. Department of Oral and Maxillofacial Medicine and Diagnostic Sciences, CWRU School of Dental Medicine - Case Western Reserve University, 9601 Chester Avenue, Cleveland, OH 44106, USA.
E-mail address: azs16@case.edu

Dent Clin N Am 68 (2024) 375–391
https://doi.org/10.1016/j.cden.2023.10.002
0011-8532/24/© 2023 Elsevier Inc. All rights reserved.

dental.theclinics.com

Pineal gland calcification

The pineal gland is a crescent-shaped neuroendocrine gland that is located between the two hemispheres of the brain. It follows the circadian rhythm and releases serotonin in the daytime and melatonin during the nighttime. Pineal gland calcification is associated with the normal aging process. In children, pineal gland calcification may be associated with brain tumors.[1] Pineal gland calcifications larger than 9 mm and radiographic signs of an "exploded pattern" or displacing calcifications within the brain tissue should raise suspicion of a tumor.[2] On the dental cone beam imaging, pineal gland calcification is observed as a solitary, midline intracranial hyperdense entity (**Fig. 1**).

Choroid plexus calcification

Choroid plexus calcifications are often encountered as part of the normal aging process and typically found in the lateral and fourth ventricles. Radiographically, they appear as small, punctuate, paired hyperdense entities in the posterior cranial fossa and inferior to the level of the pineal gland (**Fig. 2**). Typically, these choroid plexus calcifications are age-related.[1,3]

Falx cerebri calcification

Falx cerebri calcifications are noted in the midline of the cranial cavity. They appear as a wide spectrum of radiological features ranging from linear to curvilinear hyperdensities along the falx cerebri, and they are mostly idiopathic in nature with limited clinical significance (**Fig. 3**). However, falx cerebri calcifications are associated with the nevoid basal cell carcinoma syndrome (Gorlin's syndrome).[4]

Internal carotid artery calcification/intracranial internal carotid artery calcification

Internal carotid artery calcifications (ICACs) are commonly seen in older males. Patients with chronic kidney disease have a higher prevalence of ICAC because of calcium–phosphate imbalances due to renal failure. Moreover, risk factors for ICAC include a history of stroke, smoking, high cholesterol, and cardiac disease.[5]

Atherosclerotic calcifications can be seen as hyperdensities in the extracranial carotid bifurcation and in the intracranial part of the internal carotid artery.[6] These intracranial internal carotid artery calcifications (iICACs) are found in or adjacent to the carotid canal. They can range from a "rice grain" (partially calcified) to tubular

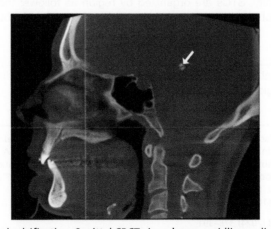

Fig. 1. Pineal gland calcification. Sagittal CBCT view shows a midline radiopacity in the posterior cranial fossa (*arrow*). (*Courtesy of* Galal Omami, BDS, Lexington, KY).

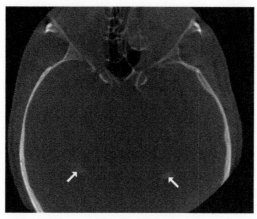

Fig. 2. Axial CBCT view shows choroid plexus calcification in the posterior cranial fossa (*arrows*). (*Courtesy of* Galal Omami, BDS, Lexington, KY).

structures (whole artery calcified) (**Fig. 4**). iICAC can occur both in the intimal and medial layer of the vascular wall.[6]

Given the associations between ICAC, stroke, and atherosclerosis, patients need to follow up with their primary care physicians after the radiographic identification of ICAC. Close monitoring and management of risk factors, such as addressing smoking cessation, controlling cholesterol, and optimizing cardiac health, are essential in these patients.[7] Moreover, patients with a history of kidney disease should receive the appropriate management to address the underlying calcium–phosphate imbalances. Health care providers can mitigate the potential complications associated with ICAC, including the stroke and atherosclerosis prognosis, by addressing these risk factors and ensuring regular medical follow-up.[8]

Vertebrobasilar artery calcification
Vertebrobasilar artery calcification (VBAC) occurs when calcium salt buildup blocks the vertebral arteries, narrowing the lumen and increasing the risk of stroke.[9] The right and

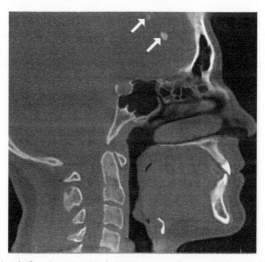

Fig. 3. Falx cerebri calcification. Sagittal CBCT image demonstrates multiple round hyperdense entities in the midline region of the anterior cranial fossa (*arrows*).

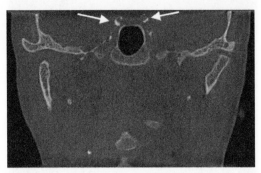

Fig. 4. Coronal CBCT view shows hyperdense entities in the parasellar region consistent with internal carotid artery calcification (*arrows*).

left vertebral arteries ascend through the foramen transversaria of the upper six cervical vertebrae; then, they merge in the posterior cranial fossa to form the basilar artery. The vertebrobasilar system supplies approximately 20% of the blood to the brain.[10]

Calcifications of the vertebrobasilar arteries can cause narrowing of lumen and lead to blood blockage, which increases the risk of strokes. VBAC is also a reliable sign of atherosclerosis and a potential risk factor for stroke. Several risk factors could contribute to VBAC formation, including old age, smoking, diabetes, hyperlipidemia, obesity, and alcohol consumption. Symptoms of VBAC may include dizziness, head/neck pain, vision loss, and spinal cord dysfunction. Patients may also experience migraines and tension headaches.[11]

VBAC is mostly noted, either unilateral or bilateral, at the level of the foramen magnum (**Fig. 5**). The shape of the calcification varies from semicircular, circular, spotty, linear, or tubular.[11] Medical management includes treating the risk factors and medical treatment. For symptomatic arterial stenoses, surgical intervention, such as endarterectomy, reconstruction, and endovascular, is the treatment of choice.[10]

Facial Skin

Osteoma cutis
Osteoma cutis (OC) is a benign soft tissue condition where osseous nodules form in the reticular dermis layer of the skin. OC is usually associated with chronic acne or dermatitis scars, as 85% of OC in body cases is believed to develop due to persistent acne.[3] Females are more frequently affected, especially during their second and third decades.

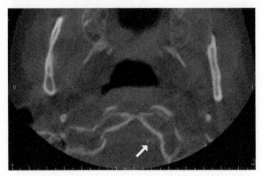

Fig. 5. Axial CBCT view demonstrates circular-shaped hyperdense entity in the foramen magnum consistent with vertebrobasilar artery calcification (*arrow*).

OC may appear to have a radiopaque outline with a radiolucent center, also described as "washer-shaped" or "donut-shaped" lesions (**Fig. 6**).[12] Treatment may vary from no treatment to surgical excisions for cosmetic purposes.[13]

Dermal filler calcification

Injectable dermal fillers are growing in popularity; however, they can result in calcifications in the soft tissues of the sites they are injected into. Calcified dermal fillers can appear as small or large (diameter >11 mm) hyperdense strands, spheres, or nodules.[14] The calcifications appear where the dermal filler was injected, and the soft tissue around them seems healthy, and they are radiographically distinguishable from bony structures close by.[15] Calcium hydroxyapatite dermal filler material may appear radiographically as spherical radiopaque calcifications.[16]

Calcification of dermal fillers appears as incidental findings on various imaging modalities, including plain radiography and CBCT.[15] Calcified dermal fillers can be diagnosed if the material is bilateral and symmetric and is distinguishable from the bone. Moreover, patients have a history of dermal filler injections.[16] Calcified dermal fillers can appear on CBCT scans as multiple, bilateral, amorphous, ring-like, or nodular radiopacities in the subcutaneous tissue (**Fig. 7**).[17] No action is needed if the dermal filler calcification is observed.[16]

Nasopharynx

Torus tubarius

Torus tubarius calcification is relatively unexplored region. In the literature, few studies have reported the calcification of the torus tubarius. Anatomically, the eustachian tube is divided into osseous, junctional, and cartilaginous portions. The calcification typically occurs in the cartilaginous portion.[18] The prevalence of torus tubarius calcification is about 0.6%.[19] Large field-of-view CBCT scans can capture the torus tubarius region. Torus tubarius calcification may be either complete or partial and they as conical hyperdensities in the cartilaginous portions of the eustachian tubes (**Fig. 8**).[18]

Maxillary Sinus

Antrolith

An antrolith is a calcified mass within the maxillary sinus.[20] It occurs due to accumulation of the mineral salts around a nidus such as a foreign body, mucus plug, or

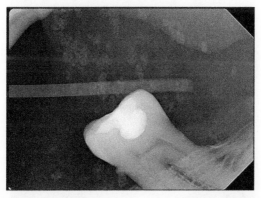

Fig. 6. Osteoma cutis. Bitewing radiograph showing multiple radiopaque calcifications in the cheek.

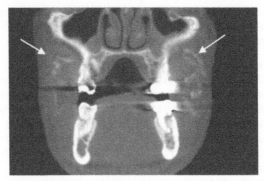

Fig. 7. Dermal fillers. Coronal CBCT image revealing multiple, amorphous radiopacities in the bilateral cheek regions (*arrows*).

microbial debris. Antroliths are typically asymptomatic and are noted as incidental findings on dental imaging. Small antroliths usually require no treatment.[20] Lesions appear as solitary or multiple radiopaque masses within the maxillary sinus, they have a wide of spectrum of radiographic presentation (**Fig. 9**).

Nasal Region

Rhinolith
A rhinolith consists of a mineralized deposit makeup surrounding a nidus in the nasal cavity. Rhinoliths are common in pediatric populations, and they typically arise from exogenous routes such as foreign body. Occasionally, patients present with symptoms of unilateral chronic purulent rhinorrhea or nasal obstruction.[21]

Rhinoliths appear as heterogeneous, irregular, hyperdense masses (**Fig. 10**). CBCT imaging is preferred over 2D imaging modalities. Patients should be referred to an ENT specialist for management.[22]

Perimandibular Region

Sialoliths
Sialoliths are calcified deposits in salivary glands. They are the most commonly occurring disease of salivary glands.[23] The etiology of these calcific deposits is the

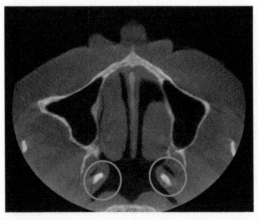

Fig. 8. Coronal CBCT image shows bilateral calcification of the torus tubarius (circles).

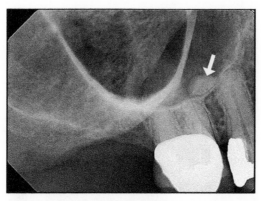

Fig. 9. The right maxillary periapical molar view demonstrates an antrolith in the floor of the maxillary sinus (*arrow*).

precipitation of calcium phosphate around desquamated epithelial cells, bacterial debris, foreign body, or mucus plug.[24] About 85% of sialoliths occur in the submandibular glands, and about 85% of submandibular gland stones arise within Wharton's duct. Symptoms of sialoliths include swelling and pain experienced during mealtimes due to salivary stimulation.[24]

Radiographically, sialoliths are usually seen as smooth, homogeneously radiopaque lesions, with evidence of multiple layers of calcification (laminated appearance) (**Fig. 11**). They can be solitary or multiple. Salivary stones are occasionally superimposed over the mandible on panoramic radiographs (**Fig. 12**). Therefore, it is recommended that cross-sectional imaging (eg, CBCT) is used to confirm the diagnosis. Small sialoliths may be managed manually by milking the gland and duct. If the stones are large and could not be negotiated through the duct, a minimally invasive surgery such as sialendoscopy may be required.[25]

Phlebolith
Phleboliths are calcified thrombi often occurring in head and neck venous malformations. Approximately 40% of all venous malformations occur in the head and neck region.[26] The calcifications may also be associated with hemangiomas. Phleboliths are frequently found in the retromandibular region and infratemporal fossa due to calcifications in the facial vein and pterygoid venous plexus.[27]

Radiographically, phleboliths appear as multiple, round, or oval, calcified bodies (**Fig. 13**). They usually have the appearance of concentric radiopaque layers (bull's

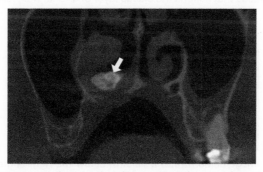

Fig. 10. Coronal CBCT image shows a rhinolith in the right nasal fossa (*arrow*).

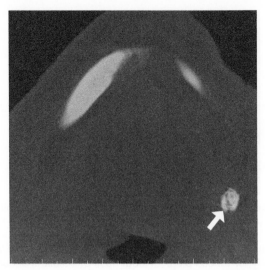

Fig. 11. CBCT view showing a sialolith in the left submandibular fossa (*arrow*).

eye or targetoid appearance).[27] MR imaging is the modality of choice for evaluating vascular lesions and associated calcifications.[26]

Tonsilloliths

Tonsilloliths occurs as a result of deposition of mineralized material in long-standing, chronically inflamed tonsillar tissues, more commonly the pharyngeal tonsils.[12,28] Patients may be asymptomatic, or they may have sore throat, irritable cough, dysphagia, otalgia, or chronic halitosis.[29]

On the panoramic radiograph, tonsilloliths may appear as single or multiple clustered, small radiopacities near the anterior border of the oropharyngeal airway space and the middle or lower one-third of the mandibular ramus (**Figs. 14** and **15**).[12,29]

Because tonsilloliths are usually asymptomatic, no treatment is required for most cases. If the patient has symptoms, tonsilloliths may be removed by curettage. Tonsillectomy may be considered for cases associated with chronic tonsillitis.[28]

Medial artery calcification (Mönckeberg atherosclerosis)

Medial artery calcification (MAC) is a non-inflammatory disease caused by vascular calcification that occurs in the tunica media layer of the wall of medium-sized arteries.[30,31] It is a degenerative process that stiffens the elastic layer of arterial wall, followed by calcium

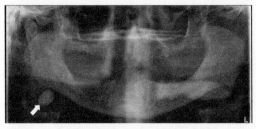

Fig. 12. Panoramic image demonstrates a sialolith below the right angle of the mandible (*arrow*). Note the laminated appearance of the lesion.

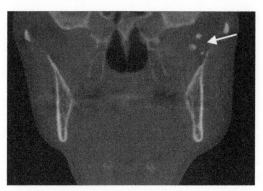

Fig. 13. Phleboliths. Coronal CBCT image reveals multiple hyperdense round entities in the left infratemporal fossa region (*arrow*).

deposition. In contrast to intimal artery calcification, the deposits do not narrow the arterial lumen and consequently do not interfere with arterial flow. The etiology of MAC is not fully known, but it is related most notably to aging, diabetes, and chronic kidney disease.[32,33] Although patients with MAC can be asymptomatic, the condition is associated with increased cardiovascular mortality and local ischemia.[34]

MAC is commonly found in muscular arteries of small to medium size, often in the lower limbs and less so in the upper extremity vessels. MAC has also been reported in renal, splenic, coronary, peripheral, and visceral arteries.[33]

MAC involving the facial (**Fig. 16**) and lingual arteries may appear on dental imaging. It appears as a straight or tortuous path of a "pipe stem" or "tram-track" pattern of calcification in the perimandibular region.[30,33]

Patients with MAC should be referred to their primary care physician for evaluation for peripheral vascular disease. The patient's cardiovascular health should also be observed due to the increased risk of cardiovascular events associated with MAC.[34]

Neck Region

Calcified carotid artery atheroma

In the United States, strokes are the fifth largest cause of death, and about 800,000 people die yearly.[35] Atherosclerotic plaques in the carotid artery are seen in 50% of stroke patients and are more common in females. Calcified carotid artery atheroma (CCAA) usually is discovered as an incidental finding on panoramic and CBCT images. For this reason, dentists should be proactive and referred patients with CCAA to their physicians for further investigation and management.[36]

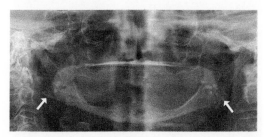

Fig. 14. Dystrophic calcifications of the palatine tonsils. Panoramic image demonstrating multiple, clustered radiopacities overlapping the posterior aspect of the ramus bilaterally (*arrows*).

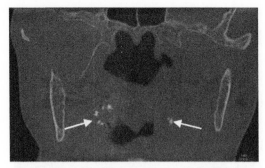

Fig. 15. Coronal CBCT image showing dystrophic calcifications in the palatine tonsils (*arrows*).

CCAAs are typically caused by calcium deposits in the tunica intima layer of the carotid artery due to accumulation of LDL cholesterol in the body. CCAAs have been associated with an increased risk of cardiovascular incidence and/or ischemic heart disease.[3,37] They are also associated with conditions, such as diabetes, hypercholesterolemia, genetic disease, sleep apnea, and disturbances of calcium metabolism.[38]

Radiographically, CCAAs may appear as either unilateral or bilateral, irregular, heterogeneous hyperdense semicircular entities located lateral to the hyoid and anteromedial to sternocleidomastoid muscle (**Fig. 17**. Occasionally, the calcification pattern may show a vertical linear distribution.[39] On panoramic images, the calcifications typically appear at the carotid bifurcation area, posteroinferior to the angle of the mandible and adjacent to the cervical vertebrae at the C3–C4 level and hyoid bone (**Fig. 18**).[33] Carotid artery calcifications may appear similar to other calcifications, such as triticeous cartilage calcification, phleboliths, and calcified lymph nodes. The diagnosis for CCAA should be made with duplex ultrasonography or angiography to determine the degree of arterial stenosis.[40]

Acute calcific tendinitis of the longus colli

The longus colli is a paired muscle that sits anterior to the cervical vertebral and spans from C1 to C3.[41] Rarely, the longus colli can become calcified when calcium hydroxyapatite deposits in the muscle's tendons, which causes a benign condition that incites

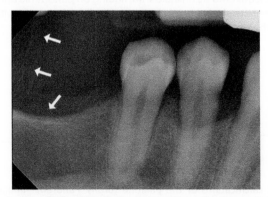

Fig. 16. Medial arterial calcification. Periapical radiograph demonstrating "tram-track" appearance of the facial artery (*arrows*).

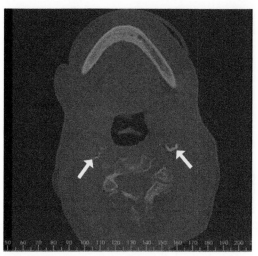

Fig. 17. Axial CBCT view shows semicircular hyperdensities in the carotid bifurcation region, consistent with calcified carotid artery atheroma (*arrows*).

a reactive aseptic inflammatory response in the body. Acute calcific tendinitis of the longus colli (ACTLC) is often known as prevertebral calcific tendinitis or retropharyngeal calcific tendinitis. It usually presents with a triad of symptoms, including odynophagia, neck stiffness, and acute onset of neck pain.[42]

ACTLC can be diagnosed on plain radiographs or CT; however, CT is the gold standard for the diagnosis. ACTLC appears as irregular or round calcifications anterior to the cervical vertebrae at C1–C2 level, typically anterior to atlas (C1) where the superior oblique tendon of the longus colli has its insertion point (**Fig. 19**).[43,44]

ACTLC is a self-limiting condition that often resolves on its own after 1 to 2 weeks.[45] The treatment of choice is nonsteroidal anti-inflammatory drugs (NSAIDs) and possible neck mobilization. Systemic corticosteroids may be used in severe cases.[43] Owing to its rare nature, ACTLC is often misdiagnosed as a retropharyngeal abscess, which entails a more invasive treatment.[43] However, ACTLC is distinguishable from retropharyngeal abscesses by the presence of a non-ring enhancing fluid collection in the prevertebral space, the absence of suppurative inflammatory retropharyngeal lymph nodes, and the presence of calcifications in the longus colli muscle.[46] It is also vital to distinguish ACTLC from other similarly presenting conditions, including meningitis, deep neck space infection, vertebral fractures, and cervical disc herniation, to avoid unnecessary invasive procedures and antibiotics.[47]

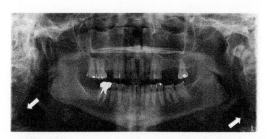

Fig. 18. Panoramic radiograph shows bilateral calcified carotid artery atheroma (*arrows*).

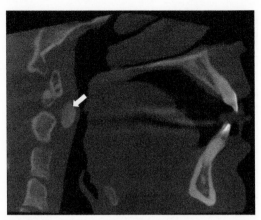

Fig. 19. Sagittal CBCT view demonstrates calcific tendinitis of the longus colli muscle (*arrow*).

Calcified lymph nodes

Calcified lymph nodes in the head and neck region are rare, occurring in only about 1% of enlarged nodes.[48] As the calcification of nodes is atypical, the mere presence of nodal calcification indicates lymph node disease.[49] Nodal calcification is common in granulomatous diseases such as sarcoidosis and tuberculosis.[49] Tuberculous lymphadenitis is thought to be the most prevalent disease associated with the dystrophic calcification of sclerotic lymph nodes.[50] The most commonly involved nodes are the submandibular, submental, superficial, and deep cervical lymph nodes.

Radiographically, calcified lymph nodes appear as multiple radiopacities with irregular "cauliflower-like" appearance along the course of a nodal chain below the inferior mandibular border or near the angle or ramus of the mandible (**Fig. 20**). Occasionally, the calcified node has a laminated pattern. Eggshell-type calcifications have been reported in silicosis, sarcoidosis, tuberculosis, and amyloidosis.

A calcified submandibular lymph node is sometimes mistaken for a submandibular salivary stone. If painful swelling accompanies a calcified submandibular mass, this strongly indicates a sialolith. Moreover, a sialolith usually has a smooth outline, whereas a calcified lymph node is usually "cauliflower-shaped", giving the impression

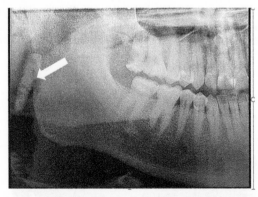

Fig. 20. Cropped panoramic radiograph demonstrates calcified lymph nodes behind the ramus of the mandible (*arrows*). (*Courtesy of* Ira Levenson, DDS, OH.)

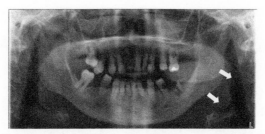

Fig. 21. Panoramic radiograph shows stylohyoid ligament calcification on the left side (*arrows*).

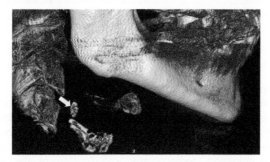

Fig. 22. 3D volume-rendered image demonstrates triticeous cartilage calcification (*arrow*).

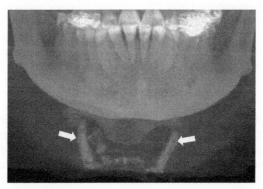

Fig. 23. 3D maximum intensity projection image demonstrates calcification of the superior cornu of thyroid cartilage (*arrows*).

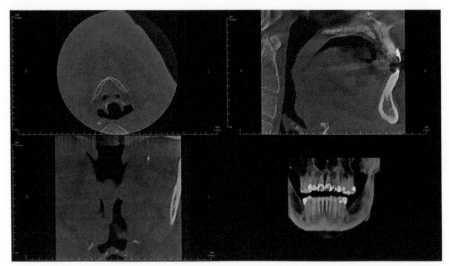

Fig. 24. CBCT volume reveals a patchy soft tissue calcification in the epiglottis.

of a collection of irregular masses. A history of tuberculosis or other disease associated with chronic lymphadenitis favors the diagnosis of calcified lymph nodes.

Stylohyoid ligament calcification
Calcification or ossification of the stylohyoid ligament is a frequent incidental finding on radiographs. The mere existence of the stylohyoid ligament complex does not ipso facto result in confirmed diagnosis of the Eagle's syndrome. The symptoms of Eagle's syndrome could range from mild discomfort to the acute neurologic and referred pain.[51]

Radiographic examination demonstrates calcification of the styloid ligament extending from the styloid process to the hyoid bone often interrupted with pseudoarthrosis.[52] The calcification can be partial or complete (**Fig. 21**).

Laryngeal calcifications
Laryngeal calcifications may involve several anatomic structures within the larynx, such as epiglottis, triticeous cartilage, and superior cornu of thyroid cartilage.

Triticeous cartilages are small round to ovoid structures embedded in the thyrohyoid ligament at the level of C3–C4 region. Although the role of the triticeous cartilage is unclear, it often gets calcified (**Fig. 22**). Calcified superior cornu of thyroid cartilage appears as linear or tubular hyperdensities on imaging. **Fig. 23** depicts the bilateral calcification of the thyroid cartilage. It may be indicative of age-related changes or underlying pathologic conditions. Calcifications of the epiglottis may appear as linear or patchy hyperdense entities (**Fig. 24**).

SUMMARY

STCs are broad category of mostly benign lesions frequently encountered by radiologists. Although STCs of the head and neck are common, not all are pathologic, therefore, only some of which may need further treatment. This review guides clinicians and radiologists to make relevant referrals and eliminate unnecessary medical referrals. By using the appropriate radiographic modality, clinicians can be informed and familiarized with recognizing STCs in the head and neck region, which can reduce anxiety and eliminate unnecessary medical expenditures for patients.

CLINICS CARE POINTS

- Head and neck soft tissue calcifications may be indicative of underlying systemic conditions (kidney disease, cardiovascular disease), and managing the underlying conditions plays an important role.
- The imaging studies can aid in determining the nature of the calcifications and guide further in the management.
- Benign clacifcations may not requre treatment.
- Stratify patients based on the risk factors.

DISCLOSURE

The author declares that he has no conflict of interest.

REFERENCES

1. Junemann O, Ivanova AG, Bukreeva I, et al. Comparative study of calcification in human choroid plexus, pineal gland, and habenula. Cell Tissue Res 2023;393(3): 537–45.
2. Doyle AJ, Anderson GD. Physiologic calcification of the pineal gland in children on computed tomography: prevalence, observer reliability and association with choroid plexus calcification. Acad Radiol 2006;13(7):822–6.
3. Singer SR, Kim IH, Creanga AG, et al. Physiologic and Pathologic Calcifications of Head and Neck Significant to the Dentist. Dent Clin North Am 2021;65(3): 555–77.
4. Kimonis VE, Singh KE, Zhong R, et al. Clinical and radiological features in young individuals with nevoid basal cell carcinoma syndrome. Genet Med 2013;15(1): 79–83.
5. Shen Y, Dong Z, Xu G, et al. Correlation between intracranial carotid artery calcification and prognosis of acute ischemic stroke after intravenous thrombolysis. Front Neurol 2022;13:740656.
6. Gocmen R, Arsava EM, Oguz KK, et al. Atherosclerotic intracranial internal carotid artery calcification and intravenous thrombolytic therapy for acute ischemic stroke. Atherosclerosis 2018;270:89–94.
7. de Weert TT, Cakir H, Rozie S, et al. Intracranial internal carotid artery calcifications: association with vascular risk factors and ischemic cerebrovascular disease. AJNR Am J Neuroradiol 2009;30(1):177–84.
8. Wu XH, Chen XY, Wang LJ, et al. Intracranial artery calcification and its clinical significance. J Clin Neurol 2016;12(3):253–61.
9. Singer SR, Mupparapu M. Cone Beam Computed Tomography Detection of Extracranial Vertebral Artery (EVA) Calcification and Ectasia. Journal of Orofacial Sciences 2019;11(1):65–70.
10. Burle VS, Panjwani A, Mandalaneni K, et al. Vertebral Artery Stenosis: A Narrative Review. Cureus 2022;14(8):e28068.
11. Katada K, Kanno T, Sano H, et al. Calcification of the vertebral artery. Am J Neuroradiol 1983;4(3):450–3.
12. Abdelkarim AZ, Lozanoff S, Abu El Sadat SM, et al. Osteoma Cutis and Tonsillolith: A Cone Beam Computed Tomography Study. Cureus 2018;10(7):e3003.

13. Hughes PSH. Multiple Miliary Osteomas of the Face Ablated With the Erbium:YAG Laser. Arch Dermatol 1999;135(4):378–80.
14. Kim GT, Lee JK, Choi BJ, et al. Malignant transformation of monostotic fibrous dysplasia in the mandible. J Craniofac Surg 2010;21(2):601–3.
15. Kwon YE, An CH, Choi KS, et al. Radiographic study of dermal fillers in the facial area: A series of 3 cases. Imaging Sci Dent 2018;48(3):227–31.
16. Valiyaparambil J, Rengasamy K, Mallya SM. An unusual soft tissue radiopacity-radiographic appearance of a dermal filler. Br Dent J 2009;207(5):211–2.
17. Mundada P, Kohler R, Boudabbous S, et al. Injectable facial fillers: imaging features, complications, and diagnostic pitfalls at MRI and PET CT. Insights Imaging 2017;8(6):557–72.
18. Syed AZ, Hawkins A, Alluri LS, et al. Rare finding of Eustachian tube calcifications with cone-beam computed tomography. Imaging Sci Dent 2017;47(4):275–9.
19. Buch K, Nadgir RN, Qureshi MM, et al. Clinical Significance of Incidentally Detected Torus Tubarius Calcification. J Comput Assist Tomogr 2017;41(5):828–32.
20. Tan YLT, Zhang Y, Chew Shen Hui B. Case report of a maxillary antrolith. Int J Surg Case Rep 2020;74:128–31.
21. Maheshwari N, Etikaala B, Syed AZ. Rhinolith: An incidental radiographic finding. Imaging Sci Dent 2021;51(3):333–6.
22. Aksakal C. Rhinolith: Examining the clinical, radiological and surgical features of 23 cases. Auris Nasus Larynx 2019;46(4):542–7.
23. Monsour PA, Romaniuk K, Hutchings RD. Soft tissue calcifications in the differential diagnosis of opacities superimposed over the mandible by dental panoramic radiography. Aust Dent J 1991;36(2):94–101.
24. Lustmann J, Regev E, Melamed Y. Sialolithiasis. A survey on 245 patients and a review of the literature. Int J Oral Maxillofac Surg 1990;19(3):135–8.
25. Adhami F, Ahmed A, Omami G, et al. Soft-tissue calcification on a panoramic radiograph: A diagnostic perplexity. J Am Dent Assoc 2016;147(5):362–5.
26. Zheng JW, Mai HM, Zhang L, et al. Guidelines for the treatment of head and neck venous malformations. Int J Clin Exp Med 2013;6(5):377–89.
27. Syed AZ, Jadallah B, Shahid K. A rare case of Phlebolith Detected by an Oral Radiologist. J Mich Dent Assoc 2018;100(5):34–8.
28. Bamgbose BO, Ruprecht A, Hellstein J, et al. The prevalence of tonsilloliths and other soft tissue calcifications in patients attending oral and maxillofacial radiology clinic of the university of iowa. ISRN Dent 2014;2014:839635.
29. Thakur JS, Minhas RS, Thakur A, et al. Giant tonsillolith causing odynophagia in a child: a rare case report. Cases J 2008;1(1):50.
30. Shahid K, Weng S, Cook L, et al. Detection of monckeberg medial sclerosis on conventional dental imaging. J Mich Dent Assoc 2017;99(3):40–2, 68–69.
31. Jensen L, Syed AZ, Odell S, et al. Mönckeberg medial arteriosclerosis in a geriatric patient with chronic kidney disease and poorly controlled diabetes reporting for a dental recall visit. Dent Clin North Am 2023;67(3):461–4.
32. Syed A, Mupparapu M. Diabetes, chronic kidney disease, hypertension, and tram-track vessels – a vicious chain. Journal of Orofacial Sciences 2022;14(2):79–80.
33. Syed AZ, Xu Y, Alluri LS, et al. Mönckeberg's medial arteriosclerosis in the oral and maxillofacial region: A pilot study. Oral Dis 2022;29(7):2938–43.
34. Lanzer P, Hannan FM, Lanzer JD, et al. Medial Arterial Calcification: JACC State-of-the-Art Review. J Am Coll Cardiol 2021;78(11):1145–65.

35. Yarnoff B, Khavjou O, Elmi J, et al. Estimating Costs of Implementing Stroke Systems of Care and Data-Driven Improvements in the Paul Coverdell National Acute Stroke Program. Prev Chronic Dis 2019;16:E134.
36. Garoff M, Ahlqvist J, Levring Jäghagen E, et al. Carotid calcification in panoramic radiographs: radiographic appearance and the degree of carotid stenosis. Dentomaxillofacial Radiol 2016;45(6):20160147.
37. Bengtsson VW, Persson GR, Berglund J, et al. Carotid calcifications in panoramic radiographs are associated with future stroke or ischemic heart diseases: a long-term follow-up study. Clin Oral Invest 2019;23(3):1171–9.
38. Amann K. Media calcification and intima calcification are distinct entities in chronic kidney disease. Clin J Am Soc Nephrol 2008;3(6):1599–605.
39. Christou P, Leemann B, Schimmel M, et al. Carotid artery calcification in ischemic stroke patients detected in standard dental panoramic radiographs - a preliminary study. Adv Med Sci 2010;55(1):26–31.
40. Schroder AGD, de Araujo CM, Guariza-Filho O, et al. Diagnostic accuracy of panoramic radiography in the detection of calcified carotid artery atheroma: a meta-analysis. Clin Oral Invest 2019;23(5):2021–40.
41. Kaplan MJ, Eavey RD. Calcific tendinitis of the longus colli muscle. Ann Otol Rhinol Laryngol 1984;93(3 Pt 1):215–9.
42. Bannai T, Seki T, Shiio Y. A pain in the neck: calcific tendinitis of the longus colli muscle. Lancet 2019;393(10185):e40.
43. Ko-Keeney E, Fornelli R. Acute Calcific Tendinitis of the Longus Colli: Not All Retropharyngeal Fluid is an Abscess. Ear Nose Throat J 2022;101(2):78–80.
44. Kim YJ, Park JY, Choi KY, et al. Case reports about an overlooked cause of neck pain: calcific tendinitis of the longus colli: Case reports. Medicine (Baltim) 2017; 96(46):e8343.
45. Ring D, Vaccaro AR, Scuderi G, et al. Acute calcific retropharyngeal tendinitis. Clinical presentation and pathological characterization. J Bone Joint Surg Am 1994;76(11):1636–42.
46. Ellika SK, Payne SC, Patel SC, et al. Acute calcific tendinitis of the longus colli: an imaging diagnosis. Dentomaxillofacial Radiol 2008;37(2):121–4.
47. Zibis AH, Giannis D, Malizos KN, et al. Acute calcific tendinitis of the longus colli muscle: case report and review of the literature. Eur Spine J 2013;22(Suppl 3): S434–8.
48. Wu G, Sun X, Ni S, et al. Typical nodal calcifications in the maxillofacial region: a case report. Int J Clin Exp Med 2014;7(9):3106–9.
49. Eisenkraft BL, Som PM. The spectrum of benign and malignant etiologies of cervical node calcification. AJR Am J Roentgenol 1999;172(5):1433–7.
50. Muto T, Michiya H, Kanazawa M, et al. Pathological calcification of the cervicofacial region. Br J Oral Maxillofac Surg 1991;29(2):120–2.
51. Gupta A, Aggrawal A, Setia P. A rare fatality due to calcified stylohyoid ligament (Eagle syndrome). Med Leg J 2017;85(2):103–4.
52. Saccomanno S, Quinzi V, D'Andrea N, et al. Traumatic Events and Eagle Syndrome: Is There Any Correlation? A Systematic Review. Healthcare 2021;9(7):825.

Imaging of Maxillofacial Injuries

Galal Omami, BDS, MSc, MDentSc, FRCD(C), Dip. ABOMR[a],*,
Barton F. Branstetter IV, MD[b]

KEYWORDS

- Mandibular fractures • Maxillofacial injuries • Radiography • Computed tomography

KEY POINTS

- The diagnosis of facial fractures usually is accomplished by a combination of clinical and imaging examinations.
- An understanding of the anatomically relevant and surgically accessible facial buttresses is critical for accurate diagnosis and proper patient management.
- Plain films will often provide adequate information for assessing mandibular and dentoalveolar fractures.
- Computed tomography (CT) is the imaging modality of choice for the evaluation of midface trauma because it allows for an accurate identification and characterization of fractures and associated sequelae.
- Careful attention should be paid to visualized portions of the skull base and cervical spine when a facial fracture is identified on CT.

INTRODUCTION

Various forms of maxillofacial injury occur in approximately 25% of trauma patients.[1] The most common causes of maxillofacial injuries are motor vehicle accidents, interpersonal violence, falls, and sports-related injuries. Complications of facial trauma include hemorrhage, infection, malocclusion, neurologic deficits, sinus drainage obstruction, airway compromise, cerebrospinal fluid leak, and ophthalmologic injury.

Imaging examinations play a crucial role in the diagnosis of maxillofacial injuries. In this regard, multidetector computed tomography (MDCT) is the imaging modality of choice for the evaluation of midface trauma because it allows for an accurate identification and characterization of fractures and associated sequelae.[1–4] A routine CT examination of the face includes helical axial 1 mm slices with coronal and sagittal reformatted images. Three-dimensional volumetric surface renderings can increase

[a] Division of Oral Diagnosis, Oral Medicine, and Oral Radiology, Department of Oral Health Practice, University of Kentucky College of Dentistry, 770 Rose Street, MN320, Lexington, KY 40536, USA; [b] Department of Radiology, University of Pittsburgh Medical Center, 200 Lothrop Street, Pittsburgh, PA 15213, USA
* Corresponding author.
E-mail address: galal.omami@uky.edu

Dent Clin N Am 68 (2024) 393–407
https://doi.org/10.1016/j.cden.2023.10.003
0011-8532/24/© 2023 Elsevier Inc. All rights reserved.

diagnostic confidence by allowing improved assessment of the spatial orientation of fractures. Most CT of the facial bone is performed without intravenous contrast and emphasizes edge-enhancing (bone) reconstructions. Panoramic imaging provides a good starting point for the initial assessment of mandibular trauma. The mandibular series of radiographs, which includes lateral oblique, posteroanterior, and reverse Towne views, can provide further information on the mediolateral displacement of mandible fractures. Dental radiographs including periapical and occlusal films are invaluable for the diagnosis of dentoalveolar fractures.

Radiographic findings that suggest a fracture of a tooth or bone include the following: (1) presence of a sharply defined 1 or 2 radiolucent lines within the anatomic boundaries of a structure, (2) loss of continuity (step deformity) in an outer border, (3) a sharp change in the level of the occlusal plane, and (4) an increase in the radiopacity of a structure.

This article describes the most frequent fracture patterns of the maxillofacial buttresses and reviews the radiographic evaluation of facial trauma.

Facial Buttresses

The facial skeleton can be conceptualized as being formed by vertical and horizontal buttresses (**Fig. 1**).[5] This buttress system provides stability to the facial skeleton and protects the central part of the face and redirects masticatory forces away from the central face. There are 3 vertical (sagittal) buttresses on either side of the face. These are the nasomaxillary, zygomaticomaxillary, and pterygomaxillary buttresses. The nasomaxillary buttress is composed of the anterior maxillary alveolus, lateral wall of the pyriform aperture, frontal process of the maxilla, lacrimal bone, and nasal process of the frontal bone. The zygomaticomaxillary buttress consists of the zygomatic process of the maxilla, body of the zygoma, frontal process of the zygomatic bone, and zygomatic process of the frontal bone. The pterygomaxillary buttress consists of the maxillary tuberosity and pterygoid process of the sphenoid bone. These vertical

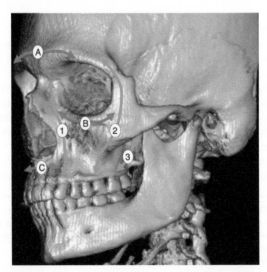

Fig. 1. Three-dimensional surface-rendered CT image in lateral oblique orientation delineates the facial buttress system. The vertical buttresses are the nasomaxillary (1), zygomaticomaxillary (2), and pterygomaxillary (3) buttresses. The horizontal components include the superior (A), middle (B), and inferior (C) buttresses.

buttresses are interconnected by 3 horizontal (axial) buttresses—the superior, middle, and inferior buttresses. The superior horizontal buttress consists of the orbital roof, cribriform plate of ethmoid bone, and superior orbital rim. The middle horizontal buttress consists of the orbital floor, inferior orbital rim, and zygomatic arches. The inferior horizontal buttress includes the maxillary alveolar process and hard palate. When treating midface fractures, realignment and proper reconstruction of the buttresses is important to restore function and appearance.[6]

Dentoalveolar Fractures

Trauma to the teeth will sometimes result in a fracture of the tooth itself, leaving the underlying maxillary or mandibular alveolus intact. At other times, a portion of the alveolus will be fractured along with the tooth or teeth. This latter scenario is called a dentoalveolar fracture. Dentoalveolar fractures can be the result of direct trauma to the teeth or from indirect trauma, usually from forced occlusion (eg, a blow to the chin). Falls and motor vehicle accidents are the most common events responsible for dentoalveolar injuries.[7] Direct trauma commonly causes injury to the maxillary central incisor region, particularly in school-age children. Predisposing factors include malocclusion, protruding incisors, and lip incompetence.

Trauma to the dentoalveolar complex can result in the following dental injuries: (1) crown fracture, with or without pulp exposure; (2) crown/root fracture; (3) root fracture; (4) concussion, a crush injury without loosening or displacement of the tooth; (5) subluxation, abnormal loosening without displacement of the tooth; (6) luxation, partial displacement of the tooth out of the alveolar socket; and (7) avulsion, complete displacement of the tooth out of the alveolar socket. Depending on their orientation and magnitude, traumatic forces can cause lateral luxation (displacement in lateral direction), extrusive luxation (displacement in a coronal direction), or intrusive luxation (displacement in an apical direction into the alveolar process). Most patients will also have associated soft-tissue injuries such as laceration and abrasion of the lip and gingiva.

Dentoalveolar trauma usually requires intraoral periapical and occlusal images to obtain adequate anatomic detail. Panoramic radiographs may not have the image resolution to reveal injuries involving the dentoalveolar structures. Cone-beam CT (CBCT) provides high-resolution images enabling excellent visualization of the teeth and supporting structures at significantly lower radiation dose and cost compared with MDCT.[8] The major limitations of CBCT include poor contrast resolution (images do not evaluate the soft tissue) and inferior signal-to-noise ratio. CBCT has been shown to outperform intraoral radiographs in the evaluation of traumatic dental injuries.[9]

Radiographic examinations of traumatized teeth may demonstrate the extent of injury to the root, periodontal ligament, and alveolar process. A tooth that has been concussed, subluxated, or luxated may demonstrate varying degrees of widening of the periodontal ligament space (**Fig. 2**A and B, Fig. **3**A and B). Intrusion may result in obliteration of the apical periodontal ligament space. Foreign bodies within the soft tissue of the lips or cheeks can be viewed by placing a periapical film in the vestibule and exposing it using half the normal exposure time (**Fig. 4**A and B). Foreign bodies within the tongue or floor of the mouth are best visualized on a standard mandibular occlusal image. If a tooth or a large dental fragment is missing, a radiographic examination of the chest and abdomen may be considered to ensure that the tooth has not been aspirated or swallowed.

Mandibular Fractures

Because of its U-shaped configuration and its prominence, the mandible is commonly fractured. Mandibular fractures are often bilateral or multifocal.[10] They occur nearly

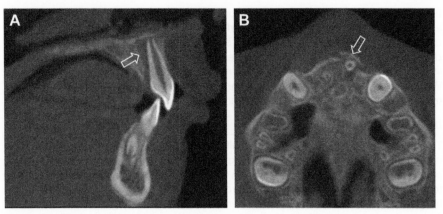

Fig. 2. Laterally luxated maxillary central incisor after a traumatic injury. Sagittal (*A*) and axial (*B*) CBCT images show partial displacement of the tooth out of its socket. Note the increase in the width of the periodontal membrane on the palatal aspect of the tooth (*arrow* in A) and fracture of the alveolar socket wall (*arrow* in B).

twice as often as midfacial fractures.[11] Mandibular fractures are classified according to the anatomic site of involvement as follows: symphysis, body, angle, ramus, condyle, coronoid process, and alveolar process. The most common mandibular fracture sites are the angle (32%), condyle (23%), body (18%), and symphysis (16%).[11] The osteology of the mandible and the presence of impacted teeth play a notable role in producing inherent structural weaknesses. Thus, fractures are seen more frequently in certain anatomic areas.

Fractures of the mandible may be classified as favorable or unfavorable, depending on the direction of the fracture line and the effect of muscle action on the fracture segments (**Fig. 5**A and B). The muscles attached to the mandible tend to further displace the bone fragments in unfavorable fractures. In favorable fractures, the muscle action tends to reduce the fragments. Condylar fractures are generally classified as intracapsular (head), extracapsular (neck), or subcondylar (base). The pull of the lateral

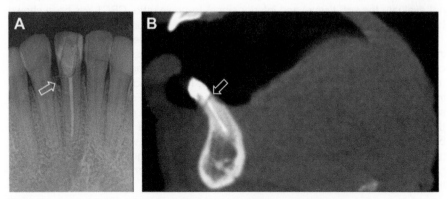

Fig. 3. Horizontal root fracture involving the mandibular central incisor. (*A*) Periapical film shows focal widening of the periodontal membrane on the lateral aspect of the tooth as an indirect sign of root fracture (*arrow*). (*B*) Sagittal CBCT image confirms the presence of root fracture (*arrow*).

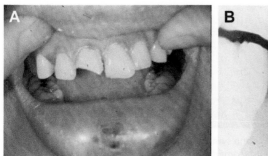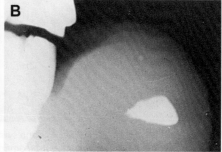

Fig. 4. (*A*) Presentation of a patient following a trauma with a crown fracture of the right permanent maxillary central incisor. (*B*) Radiographic examination of the lip revealed the tooth fragment displaced into the lower lip.

pterygoid muscle may contribute to displacement of the condylar head in an anterior and medial direction, resulting in fracture-dislocation (**Fig. 6**A and B). Bilateral fractures in the canine area can cause the mandibular symphysis to destabilize (flail mandible). This may result in posterior displacement of the tongue, which can cause partial or complete airway obstruction.

Mandible fractures can also be classified as simple (closed), compound (open), comminuted, or greenstick. A simple fracture is a complete transection of the bone with no potential sources of communication with the external environment. A fracture is regarded as compound if it communicates with the external environment, whether through skin laceration, mucosal tear, or periodontal ligament space. By definition, any fracture involving the tooth-bearing area of the jaw is a compound fracture. A comminuted fracture results in multiple fragments of bone. This type of fracture usually is the result of a high-energy impact such as a gunshot injury. Greenstick fractures, in which one cortex of bone is broken and the other is buckled, are more common in pediatric population because of the increased flexibility of the osseous structures. An

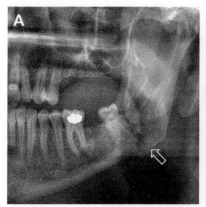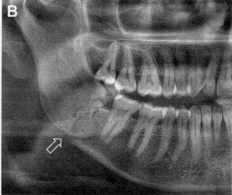

Fig. 5. Cropped panoramic images show examples of favorable (*arrow* in A) and unfavorable (*arrow* in B) fractures of the mandible. Although these fractures are similar in location, the masseter muscle is drawing the fragments together in the favorable fracture and apart in the unfavorable fracture.

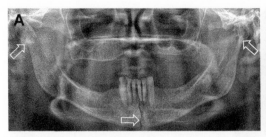
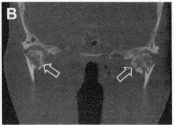

Fig. 6. (*A*) Panoramic image shows midline symphyseal and bilateral condylar fractures (*arrows*). (*B*) Coronal CBCT image shows inferomedial displacement of the condylar heads (fracture-dislocation) (*arrows*) because of unopposed action of the lateral pterygoid muscles.

oblique fracture that involves both cortical plates may appear as 2 radiolucent lines that converge at the periphery (**Fig. 7**).

Clinical signs and symptoms of mandibular fracture include malocclusion, paresthesia of the lower lip, trismus, facial asymmetry, soft tissue swelling (hemorrhage and edema), ecchymosis in the floor of the mouth, and crepitation on palpation.

Panoramic imaging, supplemented by images at 90°, such as a posteroanterior or occlusal view, provide a good initial investigation for assessing mandibular injuries. Reverse Towne view may supplement panoramic imaging, especially in cases of condylar fractures.[12] For multiple and complex fractures of the mandible, either CBCT or MDCT is the imaging modality of choice (**Fig 8**A and B).[13]

Le Fort Fractures

Le Fort fractures include a group of complex midfacial fractures that are characterized by variable degrees of craniofacial separation. These fractures were first described by René Le Fort in his series of cadaver experiments.[14] Le Fort defined the 3 weakest levels of the midfacial complex, which are classified as Le Fort I, Le Fort II, and Le Fort III fractures. Depending on the distribution of forces through the facial skeleton, the 3 fracture types can occur in combination with another, either on the same or the opposite side. By definition, the pterygoid plates are fractured in Le Fort fractures (**Fig. 9**).[5]

Le fort I fracture

Le Fort I fracture involves the anterior and lateral walls of the maxillary sinuses, nasal septum, and pterygoid plates (**Fig. 10**A–D). A sagittal palatal fracture may also be present. The fracture results in a "floating palate," which is the separation of the entire

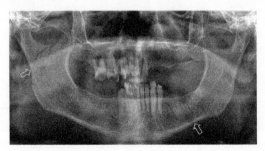

Fig. 7. Bilateral mandibular body and subcondylar fractures. Panoramic film shows what appears to be 2 fracture lines that converge at the outer border (*arrows*). The 2 lines represent an oblique fracture that involves both cortical plates.

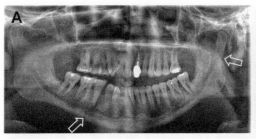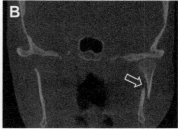

Fig. 8. Bilateral mandibular body and subcondylar fractures. (A) Panoramic radiograph shows fractures through the right body and left subcondylar region (*arrows*). Note the loss of continuity of the outer border as well as the increase in the radiopacity in the left subcondylar region caused by the overlapping of bone fragments. (B) Coronal CBCT image confirms the overlap "telescoping" of fragments (*arrow*).

palate, maxillary alveolar process, and the lower pterygoid plates from the rest of the face and skull base. The pull of the pterygoid muscles may cause displacement of the fractured segment in an inferior and posterior direction, resulting in an anterior open bite malocclusion.

Le fort II fracture

Le Fort II fracture involves the nasofrontal suture, nasal and lacrimal bones, orbital floor and inferior rims at the zygomaticomaxillary suture, maxilla, and pterygoid plates (**Fig. 11**A–D). It is also referred to as a pyramidal fracture—the apex of the pyramid is directed superiorly at the nasofrontal suture. This fracture is characterized by the separation of the nasomaxillary complex from the skull base (floating maxilla). Symptoms include bilateral periorbital edema and ecchymosis, epistaxis, infraorbital nerve paresthesia, and malocclusion.

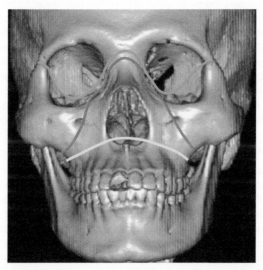

Fig. 9. Overview of Le Fort fractures. Three-dimensional surface-rendered CT image in frontal projection delineates Le Fort I ("floating palate"; yellow), Le Fort II ("pyramidal fracture"; red), and Le Fort III ("craniofacial dissociation"; green) fracture planes.

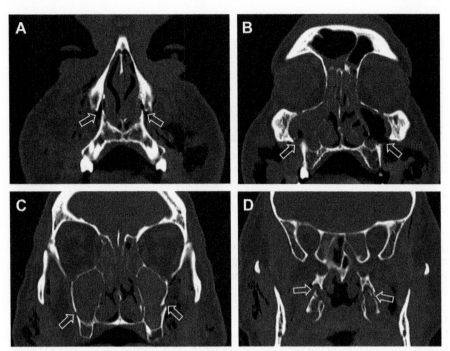

Fig. 10. Le Fort I fracture. (*A–D*) Coronal CT images in a patient with a Le Fort I injury. The fracture lines extending from just above the nasal floor, through the medial and lateral antral walls, and through the pterygoid plates (*arrows*), resulting in a "floating palate." There is bilateral antral opacification and subcutaneous emphysema.

Le fort III fracture

Le Fort III fracture causes the separation of the midfacial skeleton from the skull base. This fracture extends horizontally from the frontonasal suture through the medial orbital walls (lamina papyracea), orbital floors, and lateral orbital walls to the frontozygomatic suture and zygomatic arches (**Figs. 12**A–D and **13**A–D). A second fracture line extends from the orbital floor down the posterior maxillary sinus wall to the pterygoid plates. A "dish face" deformity is characteristic of this fracture type because of the posterior displacement of the midfacial segment. Other symptoms include cerebrospinal fluid (CSF) rhinorrhea, hemorrhage, edema, periorbital ecchymosis (raccoon eyes), infraorbital nerve paresthesia, telecanthus, epiphora, and malocclusion.

Zygomaticomaxillary Complex Fractures

Zygomaticomaxillary complex (ZMC) fractures, also known as tripod or trimalar fractures, involve disruption of the zygomatic bone in the regions of the zygomaticomaxillary, zygomaticofrontal, zygomaticosphenoid, and zygomaticotemporal sutures (**Fig. 14**). These disruptions result in varying degrees of rotation or displacement of the zygomatic bone. Patients present with pain, periorbital ecchymosis and edema, subconjunctival ecchymosis, flattening of the malar prominence, ecchymosis in the maxillary buccal sulcus, deformity at the inferior orbital rim and zygomatic buttress of the maxilla, infraorbital nerve paresthesia, and enophthalmos due to the increase in orbital volume. Limitation of mouth opening may be caused by impingement of the mandibular coronoid process against the displaced zygoma.

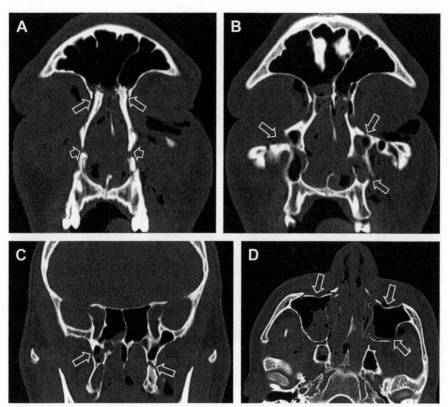

Fig. 11. Le Fort II fracture. Coronal (*A–C*) and axial (*D*) CT images demonstrate the midfacial fracture lines reflecting a Le Fort II injury (*long arrows*). Le Fort II creates a pyramid-shaped central facial fracture segment (floating maxilla). There is also orbital and subcutaneous emphysema. This patient also has Le Fort I fracture (*short arrows*).

The zygomatic bone series of radiographs include Waters, Caldwell, and submentovertex (SMV) views. Waters view is the most useful for delineating zygomatic fractures because it defines the orbital rims, orbital floor, and maxillary sinus. Caldwell view provides a good view for the zygomaticofrontal suture and lateral orbital rim. The SMV view is useful for demonstrating the status of the zygomatic arch. CT, however, is now the accepted standard of care in the evaluation of zygomatic injuries.[15] It is superior to plain films in the detection and characterization of zygomatic fractures. Additionally, CT can help demonstrate concomitant ocular injuries, hemorrhage within sinuses, subcutaneous hematoma and emphysema, and the presence of foreign bodies. Because of the high incidence of skull base and cervical spine fractures in patients with facial trauma, visualized portions of these structures should be carefully examined.[16,17]

Zygomatic Arch Fractures

Zygomatic arch fractures can occur as isolated fractures or as part of ZMC fractures (see **Fig. 14**). Isolated zygomatic arch fractures make up 10% of all zygomatic injuries, and result when a blow is applied directly to the lateral aspect of the head.[15] Characteristically, isolated fractures of the zygomatic arch result in a V-shaped or W-shaped

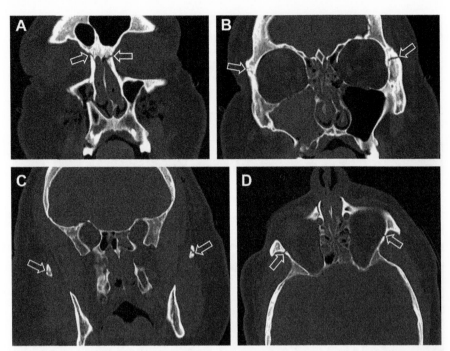

Fig. 12. Le Fort III fracture. Coronal (*A–C*) and axial (*D*) CT images in a patient with Le Fort III fracture. The fracture involves the lateral orbital walls and the zygomatic arches (*arrows*). This fracture causes separation of the entire facial skeleton from the skull base.

fracture segments. These segments are usually displaced inwards, resulting in a dimple in the overlying skin. The fracture segments may impinge on the coronoid process or temporalis muscle and interfere with mandibular movement.

Orbital Wall Blow-out Fractures

Blow-out fractures of the orbital walls result from blunt injury to the orbit by a large object (eg, fist or baseball). The impact against the thick orbital rim transmits force to the more fragile inferior and medial orbital walls, resulting in a blow-out fracture. Typically, the orbital rim in blow-out fractures remains intact. Entrapment of extraocular muscles (eg, inferior rectus) in the fracture site and herniation of orbital contents into the underlying sinus can result in restricted ocular motility, diplopia, and enophthalmos (**Fig. 15**). Paraesthesia of the infraorbital nerve may also be present in orbital floor blow-out fractures. If the medial orbital wall is involved, there may be epistaxis. Rarely, the orbital wall fracture segments may be displaced inward into the orbit, impinging on the extraocular muscles or the globe. These fractures are referred to as blow-in fractures. The size of the displaced fragment is important to surgical decision-making, so the anteroposterior and mediolateral dimensions of the fragment should be delineated.

The diagnosis of orbital blow-out fracture may be especially difficult in pediatric patients because the more pliable bone may result in "trapdoor" fractures. In these cases, the fracture segments snap back into place but the inferior rectus muscle becomes trapped beneath the fracture line.[18] One characteristic finding in such fractures is the loss of the inferior rectus muscle in the orbit.[19] When trapdoor fracture is

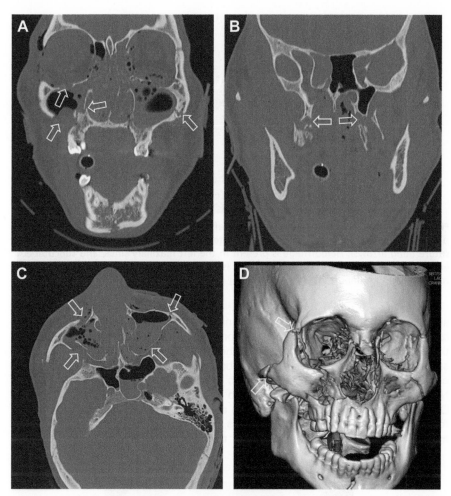

Fig. 13. Le Fort fractures. Coronal (*A* and *B*), axial (*C*), and three-dimensional surface rendering (*D*) CT images demonstrating bilateral Le Fort II and right Le Fort I and Le Fort III fractures (*arrows*). There is orbital emphysema and hemorrhage within the maxillary and ethmoid sinuses. This patient also has symphyseal and condylar fractures.

diagnosed, urgent surgical intervention is required to prevent permanent damage to the involved muscle because of ischemia.[20]

CT is the modality of choice for evaluating orbital wall fractures. It will show fractures and associated soft-tissue findings (orbital edema, subcutaneous emphysema, and antral opacification with or without an air–fluid level) with greater accuracy than plain films. If there is no bone displacement, orbital wall fractures may not be clearly identified on CT imaging but may be suspected by herniation of extraconal fat into the adjacent sinus.[21] The hemorrhage may give the herniated fat an attenuation approximating that of muscle. Thus, the diagnosis of muscle entrapment is best made clinically.

Naso-Orbital-Ethmoid Fractures

Naso-orbital-ethmoid (NOE) fractures involve the bones that form the NOE complex, including the nasal bones, medial orbital walls, ethmoid sinuses, walls of the frontal

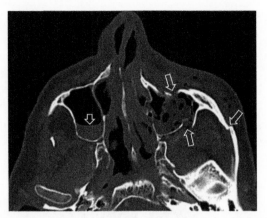

Fig. 14. ZMC fracture. Axial CT image shows a left depressed trimalar fracture. Note the displaced fractures through the anterior and posterior antral walls and zygomaticotemporal suture (*long arrows*). Hemorrhage is present in the left maxillary sinus, and subcutaneous emphysema is also present. An air-fluid level is noted in the right maxillary sinus (*short arrow*), which is an important sign of potential occult fracture.

sinuses, and cribriform plate (**Fig. 16**). The nasomaxillary and superior and middle horizontal buttresses provide structural support to this region and serve as the stabilization point for reconstruction. Just deep to the buttress system lie the thin bones and air spaces of the ethmoid sinuses. These thin bones and air-filled spaces form a so-called crumple zone, which allows the traumatic force to be dissipated. Complications of NOE fractures include telecanthus due to disruption of the medial canthal tendon, CSF leakage due to fracture through the anterior cranial fossa, enophthalmos due to comminution of the medial orbital walls, epiphora due to damage to the lacrimal apparatus, and mucocele formation due to sinus obstruction.[2] NOE fractures are

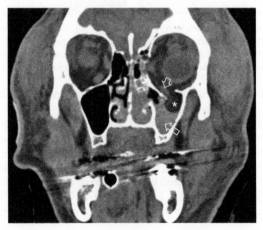

Fig. 15. Orbital floor blow-out fracture. Coronal noncontrast soft-tissue window CT image shows a blow-out fracture of the left orbital floor. Fat has herniated into the left maxillary sinus (*asterisk*), and there is partial herniation of the inferior rectus muscle (*arrowhead*). There is also blood in the in the sinus (*long arrow*).

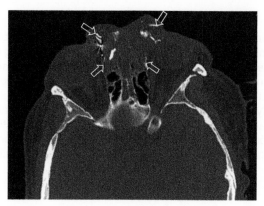

Fig. 16. NOE fracture. Axial CT scan shows severe comminution of the ethmoid region (*arrows*).

best visualized on axial CT images. Diagnosis of these fractures requires a thorough understanding of the complex anatomy of the region.

Frontal Sinus Fractures

Frontal sinus fractures represent 5% to 15% of all maxillofacial fractures.[19] They occur either as isolated fractures or as an extension of a cranial fracture. Frontal sinus fractures are generally classified by the involvement of the anterior wall (anterior table) or posterior wall (posterior table) (**Fig. 17**). Approximately two-thirds of frontal sinus fractures are limited to the anterior table. Involvement of the nasofrontal duct, degree of anterior table depression, degree of posterior table fracture, and presence of CSF leak have important implications for the surgical management of these fractures. Axial CT most clearly confirms the presence of depressed anterior wall fractures, which often are clinically obscured by overlying edema. The presence of adjacent intracranial air should be taken as evidence of fracture, even if no fracture is directly identified on imaging.

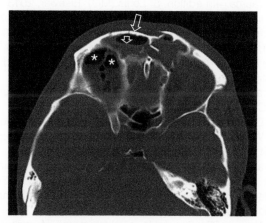

Fig. 17. Frontal sinus fracture. Axial CT image shows a depressed anterior wall fracture of the right frontal sinus (*long arrow*). There is hemorrhage within the frontal sinuses (*short arrow*). Orbital emphysema is also present (*asterisks*).

SUMMARY

The diagnosis of facial fractures usually is accomplished by a combination of clinical and imaging examinations. CT is the optimal modality for evaluating midfacial trauma and should include a high-resolution axial acquisition with multiplanar reformatted images. Three-dimensional surface renderings can increase diagnostic confidence with respect to the spatial relations of fractures. An understanding of the anatomically relevant and surgically accessible facial buttresses is critical for accurate diagnosis and proper patient management. Plain films will often provide adequate information for assessing mandibular and dentoalveolar fractures. Careful attention should be paid to visualized portions of the skull base and cervical spine when a facial fracture is identified on CT.

DISCLOSURE

The authors declare that they have no conflict of interest.

REFERENCES

1. Papageorge MB, Oreadi D. Radiographic evaluation of facial injuries. In: Fonseca RJ, Walker RV, Baxter HD, et al, editors. Oral and maxillofacial trauma. 4th edition. St Louis (MO): Elsevier; 2013. p. 232–47.
2. Winegar BA, Murillo H, Tantiwongkosi B. Spectrum of critical imaging findings in complex facial skeletal trauma. Radiographics 2013;33(1):3–19.
3. Uzelac A, Gean AD. Orbital and facial fractures. Neuroimaging Clin North Am 2014;24(3):407–24.
4. Mehta N, Butala P, Bernstein MP. The imaging of maxillofacial trauma and its pertinence to surgical intervention. Radiol Clin North Am 2012;50(1):43–57.
5. Hopper RA, Salemy S, Sze RW. Diagnosis of midface fractures with CT: what the surgeon needs to know. Radiographics 2006;26(3):783–93.
6. Fattahi T. Surgical anatomy of the maxillary region. Atlas Oral Maxillofac Surg Clin North Am 2007;15(1):1–6.
7. Reynolds JS, Reynolds MT, Powers MP. Diagnosis and management of dentoalveolar injuries. In: Fonseca RJ, Walker RV, Baxter HD, et al, editors. Oral and maxillofacial trauma. 4th edition. St Louis (MO): Elsevier; 2013. p. 248–92.
8. Cohenca N, Silberman A. Contemporary imaging for the diagnosis and treatment of traumatic dental injuries: a review. Dent Traumatol 2017;33(05):321–8.
9. Patel S, Puri T, Mannocci F, et al. Diagnosis and Management of Traumatic Dental Injuries Using Intraoral Radiography and Cone-beam Computed Tomography: An In Vivo Investigation. J Endod 2021;47(6):914–23.
10. Escott EJ, Branstetter BF. Incidence and characterization of unifocal mandible fractures on CT. AJNR Am J Neuroradiol 2008;29(5):890–4.
11. Smith BM, Deshmukh AM, Barber HD, et al. Mandibular fractures. In: Fonseca RJ, Walker RV, Baxter HD, et al, editors. Oral and maxillofacial trauma. 4th edition. St Louis (MO): Elsevier; 2013. p. 293–330.
12. Lam EWN. Trauma. In: White S, Pharoah M, editors. Oral radiology: principles & interpretation. 7th edition. St Louis (MO): Elsevier; 2014. p. 563–81.
13. De Foer B, Bernaerts A, Dhont K, et al. Facial and dental trauma. Semin Musculoskelet Radiol 2020;24(5):579–90.
14. Morris CD, Tiwana PS. Diagnosis and treatment of midface fractures. In: Fonseca RJ, Walker RV, Baxter HD, et al, editors. Oral and maxillofacial trauma. 4th edition. St Louis (MO): Elsevier; 2013. p. 416–50.

15. Ellis E. Fractures of the zygomatic complex and arch. In: Fonseca RJ, Walker RV, Baxter HD, et al, editors. Oral and maxillofacial trauma. 4th edition. St Louis (MO): Elsevier; 2013. p. 354–415.
16. Slupchynskyj OS, Berkower AS, Byrne DW, et al. Association of skull base and facial fractures. Laryngoscope 1992;102:1247–50.
17. Mithani SK, St Hilaire H, Brooke BS, et al. Predictable patterns of intracranial and cervical spine injury in craniomaxillofacial trauma: analysis of 4786 patients. Plast Reconstr Surg 2009;123:1293–301.
18. Bitar G, Touska P. Imaging in trauma of the facial skeleton and soft tissues of the neck. Br J Hosp Med 2020;81(6):1–15.
19. Fraioli RE, Branstetter BF 4th, Deleyiannis FW. Facial fractures: beyond Le Fort. Otolaryngol Clin North Am 2008;41(1):51–76.
20. Grant JH 3rd, Patrinely JR, Weiss AH, et al. Trapdoor fracture of the orbit in a pediatric population. Plast Reconstr Surg 2002;109(2):482–9.
21. Rosenbloom L, Delman BN, Som PM. Facial fractures. In: Som PM, Curtin HD, editors. Head and neck imaging. 5th edition. St. Louis, MO: Mosby; 2011. p. 491–524.

Radiographic Orofacial Findings of Systemic Diseases

Adepitan A. Owosho, DDS, DABOMP, FAAOM[a],*,
Sarah E. Aguirre, DDS, MS, DABOMP[a], Adeyinka F. Dayo, BDS, MS[b],
Temitope T. Omolehinwa, BDS, DMD, DScD, DABOM[b],
Werner H. Shintaku, DDS, MS, MS, DABOMR[a]

KEYWORDS

- Syndromes • Malignancies • Autoimmune diseases • Endocrine diseases
- Benign fibroosseous lesions • Hematologic diseases
- Dental radiographic anomalies

KEY POINTS

- Many systemic diseases have orofacial manifestations with radiographic findings.
- The dentist should be aware of the orofacial manifestations of systemic diseases to refer affected patients for appropriate diagnosis and management.
- Orofacial manifestations of systemic diseases may be the first presenting sign that leads to the initial diagnosis.

INTRODUCTION

Many systemic diseases have orofacial manifestations with radiographic findings. In this article, a range of systemic diseases with radiographic orofacial manifestations are reviewed. The systemic diseases are grouped into the following: autoimmune diseases, endocrine diseases, bone diseases, hematologic diseases, syndromes, and malignancies. The authors hope that this review article may serve as a reference document for practicing dentists.

Autoimmune Diseases

Systemic sclerosis (scleroderma)

Systemic sclerosis (SS) is a rare and complex autoimmune disease affecting the connective tissue, primarily in women.

[a] Department of Diagnostic Sciences, College of Dentistry, The University of Tennessee Health Science Center, Memphis, TN, USA; [b] Department of Oral Medicine, School of Dental Medicine, University of Pennsylvania, PA, USA
* Corresponding authors. 875 Union Avenue, Memphis, TN.
E-mail address: aowosho@uthsc.edu

Dent Clin N Am 68 (2024) 409–427
https://doi.org/10.1016/j.cden.2023.10.004
0011-8532/24/© 2023 Elsevier Inc. All rights reserved.

Clinical features. Affected patients present with tissue fibrosis, vasculopathy, usually noted as Raynaud phenomenon, and immune dysregulation. Multiple organ systems can be affected, with patients exhibiting renal crisis, pulmonary hypertension, and interstitial lung disease. Soft tissue fibrosis of the oral orifice, causing limited mouth opening, is a common finding and can also involve the masseter muscle and tongue.

Radiographic features. Mandibular osteolysis is noted in SS, which can affect the regions of muscle attachment, such as the condyles and coronoid process or mandibular angles (**Fig. 1**). Uniform widening of the lamina dura space can also be observed on both computed tomography (CT) and periapical radiographs. T2-weighted MRI will show low signal intensity in areas of soft tissue fibrosis. Ultrasounds show echogenicity in areas of soft tissue fibrosis.[1]

Endocrine Diseases

Diabetes mellitus

Diabetes mellitus (DM) is a chronic metabolic disorder leading to hyperglycemia, caused by either abnormal insulin secretion or action or both.[2] In Type 1 DM, pancreatic B-cell destruction leads to absolute insulin deficiency, hence the need for daily insulin injections to control blood glucose levels. Type 1 DM can develop at any age but occurs most frequently in children and adolescents. Type 2 DM is more common in adults and accounts for approximately 90% of DM. It results from the inability of the body to make use of available insulin, also known as insulin resistance. DM is diagnosed, among other guidelines, as fasting plasma glucose $\geq$ 126 mg/dL ($\geq$7 mmol/L), random plasma glucose $\geq$ 200 mg/dL ($\geq$11.1 mmol/L) on two occasions, or an glycated hemoglobin (HbA1C) $\geq$ 6.5%.

Clinical features. Classical signs of polyphagia, polydipsia, and polyuria characterize DM. Other symptoms include unexplained weight loss, fatigue, blurred vision, increased hunger, and slow-healing sores. Oral manifestations of uncontrolled diabetes may include xerostomia, burning mouth, candidiasis, salivary gland enlargement, and periodontal disease. Periodontal disease is more common in people with uncontrolled DM and is considered a complication of diabetes.[3] DM is a significant risk factor associated with peri-implantitis.

Radiographic features. Periodontal disease exhibiting severe alveolar bone loss is common in uncontrolled DM patients (**Fig. 2**). Medial arterial calcification of the internal carotid arteries is frequently noted as an incidental finding on cone-beam CT (CBCT) of diabetic patients and may be an indicator of DM (**Fig. 3**).[4]

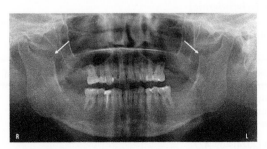

Fig. 1. Panoramic radiograph from a 32-year-old woman affected by systemic sclerosis displaying (*arrows*) bilateral coronoid process destruction.

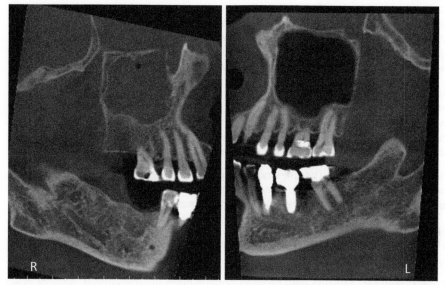

Fig. 2. Note the severe periodontal bone loss in a diabetic patient in this sagittal section CBCT.

Osteopenia and osteoporosis

Osteopenia is a metabolic bone condition resulting in an imbalance of bone deposition and resorption, leading to a net reduction in bone formation. Osteopenia is considered a normal variation because it occurs as part of aging. However, this gradual and progressive loss in bone mass may become significant, leading to osteoporosis. Although osteoporosis is diagnosed by dual X-ray photon absorptiometry, the dentist may be the first to detect signs of this condition on routine dental imaging.[5] Therefore, radiographs of postmenopausal women should be evaluated closely, as they are more at risk.[5,6] A T-score of −2.5 or below is considered osteoporosis.

Clinical features. Clinically, patients may have bone pain. Complications of osteoporosis may include bone fractures such as proximal femur, distal radius, ribs, and vertebrae.

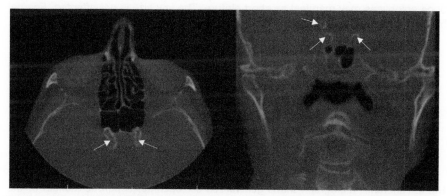

Fig. 3. Axial and coronal CBCT images showing medial arterial calcification of the intracranial internal carotid arteries as an incidental finding in a patient with type II DM.

Radiographic features. Osteopenia decreases trabeculae and bone density, which appears radiographically as thinning of the cortices, especially the inferior cortex of the mandible.[5,6] These radiographic features become increasingly prominent with progression to osteoporosis with no effect on jaw size. The teeth appear prominent against the background of the demineralized bone with thinned lamina dura (**Fig. 4**).

Hyperpituitarism/gigantism/acromegaly

Hyperpituitarism results from hyperfunction of the anterior lobe of the pituitary gland, which may result in an increased production of growth hormone.[7] This may be due to a benign secretory tumor of the somatotrophs. Acromegaly occurs in skeletally mature adults and gigantism in skeletally immature children.[7,8]

Radiographic features. There are no changes in bone density or trabeculation. However, the jaw tends to be larger in hyperpituitarism, especially the mandible. There can be hypercementosis of the premolar and molar teeth.

Hypopituitarism

Hypopituitarism results from reduced secretion of pituitary hormones, especially growth hormone.[9]

Clinical features. Patients may develop skeletal class III prognathism, anterior open bite, or an increased mandibular angle with the spacing of teeth.[7,8] It also leads to hypertrophy of soft tissue such as nose, lips, tongue (macroglossia), hands, and feet.

Radiographic features. Retained deciduous teeth, delayed eruption of permanent teeth, and agenesis of the third molars are common.

Hypoparathyroidism and pseudohypoparathyroidism

Hypoparathyroidism results from insufficient secretion of parathyroid hormone (PTH), most commonly due to unintentional damage or removal of the parathyroid glands during thyroid surgery. In pseudohypoparathyroidism, there is a defect in the response of target tissue cells to normal levels of PTH. The result of both cases is low serum levels of calcium, leading to activation of receptor activator of the nuclear factor-κB receptor on pre-osteoclasts to upregulate osteoclastic activity.[10]

Clinical features. Manifestations include tetany of the wrist and ankle joints, sensorineural abnormalities (paresthesia), parkinsonism, epilepsy, and neurologic changes such as anxiety and depression. In pseudohypoparathyroidism, early closure of bone epiphyses may manifest as short stature. The jaw size is not affected. Enamel hypoplasia and delayed tooth eruption may be seen clinically.

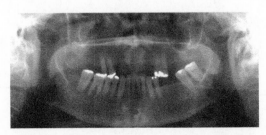

Fig. 4. Panoramic radiograph shows generalized osteopenic/osteoporotic changes of the mandible. Note the overall thinning of cortical boundaries and reduction in trabeculation. (*Courtesy of* Dr Galal Omami, Lexington, KY.)

Radiographic features. Radiographically, there may be external root resorption or dilaceration.[10]

Hyperparathyroidism

Hyperparathyroidism results from an excess of circulating PTH, which favors osteoclastic resorption of bone and mobilization of calcium from the skeleton, with an ultimate increase in serum calcium PTH and alkaline phosphatase levels. Primary hyperparathyroidism results from PTH overproduction from a benign secretory tumor of one of the parathyroid glands in about 85% of cases, whereas most of the remaining cases result from hyperplastic parathyroid glands secreting excess PTH.[8] Secondary hyperparathyroidism results from a compensatory increase in the production of PTH in response to hypocalcemia seen in cases such as renal osteodystrophy.

Clinical features. Primary hyperparathyroidism occurs mainly in adults 30 to 60 years of age and is more prevalent among females. The clinical manifestations are classically called the triad of "stones, bones, and groans," which includes renal calculi, osteoporosis, arthritis, bone fracture, and gastrointestinal symptoms such as peptic ulcers. The teeth may be hypoplastic and hypocalcified with loss of enamel. There may be gradual loosening, drifting, and loss of teeth. These features are also noted in renal osteodystrophy.[11] Giant cell lesions known as brown tumors may be noted in the bone.[8,11]

Radiographic features. The jaw size is unaffected. Bone density decreases with the bony architecture becoming granular. The calvarium has a granular appearance with the loss of diploic trabeculae and thinning of the cortices, termed "salt and pepper" skull. Loss of the lamina dura makes the roots appear tapered. Giant cell lesions may be seen as ill-defined radiolucencies.

Bone Diseases

Osteopetrosis (Albers-Schonberg disease, marble bone disease)

Osteopetrosis is an inherited bone disorder resulting from a defect in the differentiation and function of osteoclasts.[12] It is inherited in an autosomal recessive or dominant manner, referred to as osteopetrosis congenita and osteopetrosis tarda, respectively. The lack of normal functioning osteoclasts results in the failure of bone remodeling and an increase in bone density.[12] The recessive form of osteopetrosis is severe, manifests in infants, and has a fatal outcome. The benign dominant form in adults may be an incidental finding on radiographs or a case of bone fracture.

Clinical features. Bone pain and cranial nerve palsies may be a concern. In osteopetrosis, bone is fragile and susceptible to fracture and infection due to reduced vascularity from progressive loss of cancellous bone trabeculae.

Radiographic features. Increased bone density is noted as significant radiopacity and increased jaw size (**Fig. 5**).[12] Owing to the homogenous radiopacity of the alveolar process, the contrast between the cortical outline of the jawbone and the alveolar process is lost. The inferior alveolar canals appear prominent and narrowed.[12] The lamina dura is thick, and the increased radiopacity of the alveolar process obscures the perception of the roots of the teeth. The teeth are hypocalcified and prone to caries and may be missing, lost early, or malformed.[13]

Paget disease of bone (osteitis deformans)

Paget disease of bone (PDB) is a polyostotic skeletal disorder that may involve a paramyxovirus infection with subsequent changes to the host cell genome. It is more

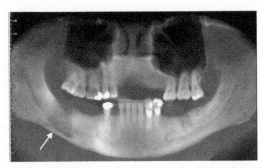

Fig. 5. Reconstructed panoramic CBCT image of a case of osteopetrosis. Note the increased radiopacity of the jaws, narrowing of the mandibular canals, and development of osteomyelitis in the body of the right mandible (*arrow*). (*Courtesy of* Dr Galal Omami, Lexington, KY.)

prevalent in men more than 65 years of age.[8,14] Mutations have been identified in *SQSTM1*, *TNFRSF11 A*, and *TNFRSF11 B*, which are genes involved in bone remodeling.[14] Abnormal osteoclasts produce bone resorption followed by a protuberant osteoblastic activity, forming poor-quality woven bone.

Clinical features. PDB often affects the pelvis, femur, vertebrae, and skull, with the maxilla being affected twice as often as the mandible. Patients with PDB may have ill-defined sensorineural pain due to the impingement of neural foramina and canals. Jaw enlargement leads to drifting of teeth, spacing, malocclusion, and ill-fitting removable prosthesis.

Radiographic features. Classically, PDB has three radiographic stages: an early stage of primarily osteoclastic activity where the bone appears radiolucent, an intermediate stage with granular bone appearing within the radiolucent areas, and the mature stage where bone becomes dense and radiopaque.[8,14] The trabeculae may be organized into round, radiopaque patches of abnormal bone, creating a cotton wool appearance.[8,14,15] The lamina dura is thinned or obscured into the changed bony pattern, and there may be hypercementosis. The specific bone pattern alterations, late age of onset, enlargement of the involved bone, and pronounced elevation of serum alkaline phosphatase aid in diagnosis.

Hematologic Diseases

Sickle cell disease
Sickle cell disease (SCD) is an inherited autosomal recessive disorder of hemoglobin. Mutation in the β-globin chain causes the formation of abnormal hemoglobin S (HbS), which alters the shape of red blood cells and interferes with the delivery of oxygen to tissues.

Clinical features. Characteristic clinical manifestations include mucosal pallor and jaundice secondary to anemia, massive hemolysis, bone pain during a sickle cell crisis, aseptic pulpal necrosis, osteomyelitis, and oral neuropathies.

Radiographic features. Bone infarcts can be noted in the mandible or temporomandibular joint (TMJs) of children with SCD and appear as hyperintensity and "rim-like enhancements" of the bone marrow in T2-weighted MR images.[16] Hypointensity is observed on T1-weighted MR images, often with cortical thinning and expansion within the medullary cavities. Panoramic and CBCT images show large spaces between the trabeculae in areas of marrow hyperplasia caused by chronic anemia (**Fig. 6**). The "hair-on-end" sign is also noted as a radiologic feature of hemolytic anemia in bone marrow hyperplasia of the skull.[17]

Thalassemia
Thalassemia is an autosomal recessive hemoglobin disorder similar to SCD.

Clinical features. The main oro-facial manifestation of thalassemia include frontal bossing, pug nose, class II malocclusion, and maxillary skeletal protrusion, giving a chipmunk-like face, high caries index, and severe gingivitis.

Radiographic features
Thinning of the bony cortex and spaces in bony trabeculae are observed radiographically as well as[18] larger bony rami and thickening of the frontal bone (**Fig. 7**). The "hair-on-end" sign in the skull is also noted in thalassemia.[17] In addition, hypoplasia or aplasia of the paranasal sinuses may be seen.

Arteriovenous malformations
Arteriovenous malformations (AVMs) may be congenital, familial, or acquired vascular lesions. They are characterized by abnormal communication/connection between arteries and veins without a capillary network serving as a connection channel. Although congenital types are more common, acquired AVMs can arise from trauma or hormonal changes. These can present in the head and neck intraosseous or soft tissue sites like the brain, spinal cord, jaws, buccal mucosa, palate, and lip.

Clinical features. AVM in the head and neck region may present as a pulsatile, compressible localized swelling that is persistent and may progressively enlarge. Patients can also present with ecchymosis or spontaneous bleeding. Life-threatening severe hemorrhage is a complication of AVM.

Radiographic features. Radiolucency, including multilocular or "soap bubble" appearance, can be seen with intraosseous jaw lesions on tomographic imaging (**Fig. 8**).[19] Imaging diagnosis can be by magnetic resonance angiography, CT, MRI, contrast-enhanced CT angiography, and ultrasound.

Syndromes

Nevoid basal cell carcinoma syndrome
Nevoid basal cell carcinoma syndrome (NBCCS), also known as Gorlin–Goltz syndrome, is an autosomal dominant disorder caused by a mutation of *PTCH1*, a tumor

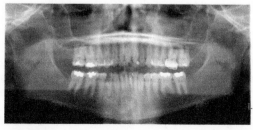

Fig. 6. Panoramic radiograph shows large trabecular spaces noted in the posterior mandible, more significant in the lower left body of mandible in the molar region of a sickle cell anemia patient. (*Courtesy of* Dr Mel Mupparapu, Professor of Oral Medicine, School of Dental Medicine, University of Pennsylvania).

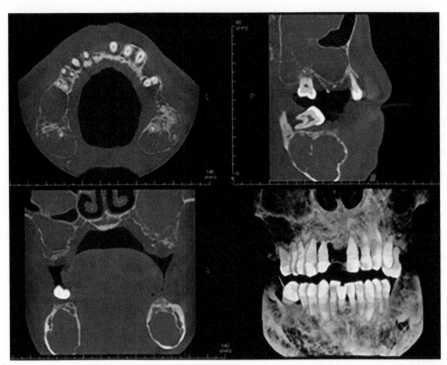

Fig. 7. CBCT multiplanar reconstruction showing generalized expansion and thinning of the lingual/palatal and buccal/labial cortices with sparse trabeculation of the alveolar process in a patient with thalassemia. (*Courtesy of* Dr Mel Mupparapu, Professor of Oral Medicine, School of Dental Medicine, University of Pennsylvania.)

suppressor gene.[20,21] NBCCS is characterized by many different clinicoradiographic features, some of which can be identified by a dentist, raising suspicion about NBCCS.

Clinical features. Clinical features are categorized into major or minor features based on the frequency of presentation in patients with this syndrome. A diagnosis of NBCCS can be made by a combination of two major features, one major feature and molecular confirmation, or one major and two minor features.[22]

Major features of NBCCS include odontogenic keratocyst (OKC) of the jaw in an individual less than 20-years-old or multiple OKCs, basal cell carcinoma in an individual less than 20-years-old or excessive numbers of basal cell carcinomas disproportionate to sun exposure, palmar or plantar pitting, calcification of the falx cerebri, a first degree relative with NBCCS, and desmoplastic medulloblastoma.[22]

Minor features of NBCCS include skeletal malformations (kyphoscoliosis, polydactyly), rib anomalies, macrocephaly, micrognathia, cleft lip/palate, meningioma, ovarian/cardiac fibroma, and lymphomesenteric cyst.[22] OKC can be the first presenting sign of this syndrome. NBCCS should be suspected with the manifestation of an OKC in a patient younger than 20 years or multiple recurrences of OKC in a young patient.[22]

Radiographic features. OKC presents as a well-defined unilocular or multilocular radiolucency in the jaws and may be associated with an unerupted tooth (**Fig. 9**). It

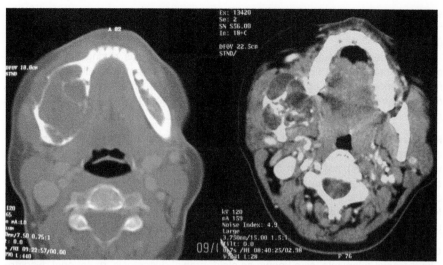

Fig. 8. CT arteriovenous (AV) malformation right (R) mandible: Axial computed tomography scans in both bone and soft tissue windows show bucco-lingual expansion with loss of bony cortex noted in the area of the lesion (right premolar–molar region).

may be solitary or multiple, with a locally destructive potential, without a tendency for buccolingual cortical expansion. Calcification of the falx cerebri can be identified on wide-field view CBCTs in dental practices.

Gardner syndrome

A variant of familial adenomatous polyposis, Gardner syndrome is an autosomal dominant disorder caused by mutation in the adenomatous polyposis coli gene, a tumor suppressor gene on chromosome 5q21.[23] It is a life-threatening condition due to its association with colorectal adenocarcinoma. As there are significant oral/dental manifestations,[24] dentists may play a role in identifying this condition.

Clinical features. Gardner syndrome is characterized by a classic triad of features comprising polyps in the colon, osteomas of the bone, including the jaws, and cutaneous and subcutaneous soft tissue tumors such as fibromas, epidermal and

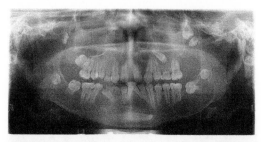

Fig. 9. Panoramic radiograph of a 15-year-old woman with nevoid basal cell carcinoma syndrome displaying multiple well-defined radiolucencies in the mandible and maxilla representing OKCs. Some are associated with impacted teeth, tooth displacement, and root resorption.

sebaceous cysts, and desmoid tumors.[25] Other oral/dental features include odontomas, supernumerary teeth, impacted and ectopic teeth, and hypercementosis (**Fig. 10**).[24]

Most patients develop hundreds of colorectal adenomas during childhood and adolescence. Without prophylactic colectomy, nearly all patients will develop colorectal adenocarcinoma by the age of 40 to 50 years.[26] Osteomas of the jaw are the most common oral/dental abnormality.[27] Orofacial features may precede colonic polyps.

Radiographic features. Osteomas present as well-defined radiopacities without the involvement of the root apices. Two distinct patterns of osteomas, focal (80%) and widespread (20%), have been described.[28] Osteomas are usually asymptomatic but can cause facial asymmetry, disfigurement, and restricted mouth opening depending on their location within the craniofacial complex.[24] The detection of three or more osteomas in the maxillofacial region suggests the syndrome.[29] Odontomas and multiple unerupted supernumerary teeth can all be identified on a radiograph.

Cleidocranial dysplasia

Cleidocranial dysplasia, also known as cleidocranial dysostosis, mutational dysostosis, or Scheuthauer–Marie–Sainton syndrome, is an autosomal dominant disorder caused by mutation of *RUNX2* on chromosome 6p21.[30,31]

Clinical features. Cleidocranial dysplasia presents with hypoplastic or aplastic clavicles, supernumerary teeth, and distinctive facial features such as midface hypoplasia, hypertelorism, and frontal bossing.[31] These dental anomalies enable dentists to play an integral role in identifying this condition (**Fig. 11**).

Radiographic features. Numerous unerupted permanent and supernumerary teeth can result in a rather chaotic picture of the dentition.

Ectodermal dysplasia

Ectodermal dysplasia (ED) represents a heterogeneous group of inherited disorders affecting ectodermal-derived tissues, including the hair, nails, teeth, skin, and sweat glands.[32] ED has varying patterns of inheritance, including X-linked recessive, autosomal dominant, or autosomal recessive.

Clinical features. Craniofacial and orodental abnormalities are frequently observed in EDs, including frontal bossing, a depressed nasal bridge, cleft palate, hypodontia, anodontia, and morphologic disturbances of the teeth.[33,34] A study of genetically

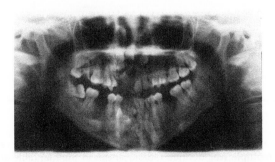

Fig. 10. Panoramic film showing multiple supernumerary and impacted teeth, odontomas, and dense bone islands throughout both jaws in a patient with Gardner syndrome.

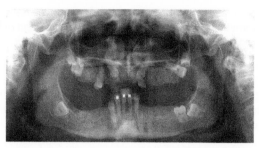

Fig. 11. Panoramic projection of a patient with cleidocranial dysplasia and several impacted and retained teeth.

confirmed X-linked ED, which included 23 males and 36 heterozygous females, showed the mean number of missing teeth to be 22 in males (range 14–28) and 4 in females (range 0–14).[35] Maxillary and mandibular lateral incisors, first premolars, and mandibular central incisors were missing in 100% of affected males.[35] The maxillary central incisors, first molars, and maxillary canines are the most stable teeth in affected males.[33,35] Abnormal crown morphology, including tapered and conical incisors, is a frequent finding in ED.[33,34,36]

Radiographic features. Missing teeth, without impaction, are observed on dental radiographs (**Fig. 12**). Taurodontism and fused roots may also be observed[35,36]

Syndromes associated with benign fibro-osseous lesions
Various syndromes are associated with the polyostotic variant of fibrous dysplasia (FD), including Jaffe-Lichtenstein syndrome (JLS), McCune–Albright syndrome (MAS), and Mazabraud syndrome (MS).[37,38] FD results from post-zygotic activating mutations of the guanine nucleotide binding protein, alpha stimulating (*GNAS*) gene.[37,38]

Clinical features. MS is a rare form of FD, with more than 100 reported cases, which often localizes to the lower limbs and is associated with intramuscular myxomas.[39] JLS may be used to describe polyostotic FD with café-au-lait skin pigmentation without endocrinopathies.[40] Affecting around 3% of patients with polyostotic FD, MAS is characterized by café-au-lait pigmentation and multiple endocrinopathies, often presenting as precocious puberty, thyroid abnormalities, or growth hormone excess.[37,38] Café-au-lait skin

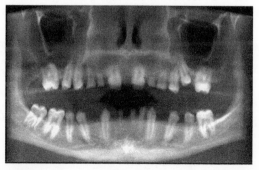

Fig. 12. Panoramic radiograph of a patient with ectodermal dysplasia showing several missing teeth. (*Courtesy of* Dr Anitha Potluri, School of Dental Medicine, University of Pittsburgh.)

pigmentation presents as tan-to-brown macules with well-defined irregular borders.[37,38,40] Asymptomatic clinical expansion is often the first sign of FD.[37] The maxilla is more frequently involved than the mandible in the head and neck.[37]

Radiographic features. The radiographic appearance of FD is classically described as having a ground-glass radiopacity with ill-defined blending borders.[37,40,41] This appearance may change over time to become more mixed and heterogeneous with age.[41] FD often expands and thins the cortices but rarely breaches them.[40,41] Sphenoid and skull base involvement are characteristic of FD.[40,41]

Malignancies

Leukemia and lymphoma

Leukemia and lymphoma, also called hematolymphoid neoplasms, are malignancies that affect the cells of the immune system at various stages of differentiation and include several subtypes. Leukemia is classified as acute lymphocytic leukemia, acute myeloid leukemia, chronic lymphocytic leukemia (CLL), and chronic myeloid leukemia.[42] Two broad categories of lymphoma are Hodgkin lymphoma (HL) and non-Hodgkin lymphoma (NHL).[43] HL progresses by contiguous nodal spread and is often localized (**Fig. 13**). NHL tends to spread hematogenously and is often systemic and extranodal. NHL is the most common type in the head and neck, with diffuse large B-cell lymphoma (DLBCL) being the most common subtype.[44,45] Burkitt lymphoma (BL) is an aggressive type of NHL that may cause facial swelling or exophytic mass in the jaws and primarily affects children.[46]

Clinical features. Leukemia is associated with anemia, thrombocytopenia, neutropenia, and altered granulocyte function.[47,48] Fatigue, fever, night sweats, and swollen lymph nodes are often observed in patients with leukemia or lymphoma, regardless of age. However, the symptoms of each condition can be distinct, depending on the type of leukemia or lymphoma and the affected structure.

Leukemia may initially manifest in the oral cavity due to leukemic cells infiltrating and reducing the normal bone marrow.[48] This typically manifests as gingival enlargement, bleeding, petechiae, and ulceration.[48–50]

When lymphoma presents intraorally, the most frequently involved sites are the gingiva, palate, tonsils, tongue, floor of the mouth, buccal mucosa, and retromolar trigone.[46,51,52] Lymphoma-associated alveolar bone loss with inflammation and pain may delay treatment because it can mimic periodontal disease.[52,53]

Radiographic features. The most common imaging finding in leukemia and lymphoma affecting the jaws is an osteolytic lesion with ill-defined margins (**Fig. 14**).[47,53–55]

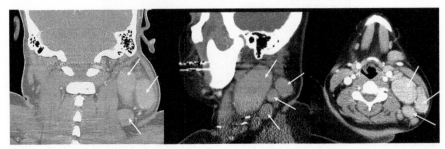

Fig. 13. Computed tomographic coronal, lateral, and axial views showing multiple enlarged, homogenous cervical nodes (*arrows*) associated with Hodgkin lymphoma.

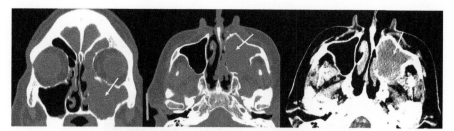

Fig. 14. Computed tomographic coronal and axial views (bone and soft tissue windows) of an atypical B-cell lymphoma in the left maxillary sinus (*arrows*).

However, DLBCL and leukemic infiltrates may be osteogenic,[47,55] and BL may have well-defined margins.[47]

Loss of lamina dura, irregular and diffuse widening of the periodontal ligament space, and floating teeth are the most common dental findings in leukemia and lymphoma.[47] Periodontal changes and periapical lesions are more common in leukemia, whereas floating teeth are more common in BL.[47]

Multiple myeloma

Multiple myeloma (MM) is a malignancy associated with the abnormal proliferation of monoclonal plasma cells in the bone marrow. MM produces excessive nonfunctional immunoglobulin and stimulates the maturation of atypical osteoclast precursors.

If metastatic diseases are excluded, MM accounts for about 50% of all bone malignancies.[56–59] The incidence of MM increases with age (median age at diagnosis is 69 years) and is more common in black males than other demographic groups.[57,58,60,61]

Clinicoradiographic features. The clinical manifestations of MM include skeletal pain, fatigue, anemia, leukopenia, thrombocytopenia, hypercalcemia, weakened immune system, and renal malfunction.[60,62,63] The acronym CRAB, which stands for hypercalcemia, renal disorders, anemia, and bone lesions, categorizes MM manifestations.[61]

The jaws are affected in about 30% of MM cases, more often in the mandible, especially in the posterior portion and jaw angle.[56,62] The presence of jaw lesions implies an unfavorable prognosis because they indicate advanced-stage disease.[62,64]

Radiographic features. MM is characterized by the presence of sharply punched-out lytic bone lesions in different parts of the skeleton, such as the skull, mandible, spine, ribs, and long bones (**Fig. 15**).[56,61,65] Reduced bone density resembling osteopenia or osteoporosis is described.[61,66] Sclerotic bone lesions, displaying well-defined areas of increased radiodensity, may also indicate MM.[59] Plasmacytomas, localized clusters of myeloma cells, can be detected as discrete masses in either bone or soft tissue, without signs of systemic disease.[59] MRI reveals abnormal bone marrow patterns, with a diffuse hypointensity on T1-weighted images, diffuse hyperintensity on T2-weighted images, and enhancement after gadolinium administration, providing important diagnostic and prognostic information.[67,68] Increased tracer uptake on bone scans and 18F-fluorodeoxyglucose PET/CT scans assist in identifying abnormal plasma cells and monitoring therapy response.[68,69]

Metastatic lesions affecting the jaws

Metastasis, or metastatic disease, happens when malignant cells from a primary site travel through the bloodstream or lymph vessels to other body regions, establishing new tumors, which are considered a separate disease from the primary tumor.[70]

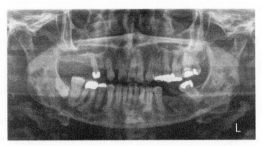

Fig. 15. Panoramic projection showing multiple small, punched-out lesions of multiple myeloma involving the mandible.

Clinicoradiographic features. Metastasis to the jaws is relatively uncommon, comprising about 1% to 8% of oral malignancies.[71,72] The posterior mandible, tongue, and TMJ are the most frequently affected sites (**Fig. 16**).[73–75] Metastases to the jaws may be associated with malignant lesions in various primary sites, including the lungs, kidneys, liver, thyroid, adrenal glands, prostate, and breast. Clinical features of metastatic diseases include ulcerated masses, swelling, pain, and paresthesia.[72,73,75] Lesions tend to be localized and affect bone more frequently than soft tissues and the mandible more than the maxilla.[70,76]

Radiographic features. A common radiographic feature is a poorly defined radiolucent lesion with irregular margins.[73,77] Metastases can be radiolucent, radiopaque, or both.[72] Additional features include cortical bulging, erosion with a "sunburst" appearance, and periosteal bone-thickening along the outer jaw surface. Root resorption is rare because malignant lesions are more prone to cause faster bone resorption.[77]

These radiographic characteristics may also manifest in nonspecific inflammatory, reactive, or hyperplastic benign lesions.[77–79] Therefore, further testing, including PET and tissue biopsy, is often indicated to confirm the diagnosis.

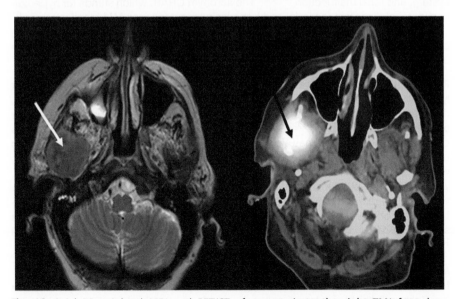

Fig. 16. Axial T2-weighted MRI and PET/CT of metastasis to the right TMJ from lung adenocarcinoma.

SUMMARY

In summary, the authors discussed the orofacial clinicoradiographic features of systemic diseases that manifest in the orofacial region. It is crucial for clinicians to be aware of these findings as they may be the first manifestation of these systemic diseases.

CLINICS CARE POINTS

- Systemic diseases may present with radiographic changes in the orofacial region.
- These radiographic findings may not be encounted regularly in a day-to-day dental practice and may be the first sign of the systemic disease.
- The radiographic orofacial features of these systemic diseases may vary from radiolucent, mixed radiopacities to complete radioopaque appearances.

DISCLOSURE

All authors declare that there are no financial conflicts associated with this study and that the funding source has no role in conceiving and performing the study.

REFERENCES

1. Abdel Razek AA. Imaging of connective tissue diseases of the head and neck. NeuroRadiol J 2016;29(3):222–30.
2. Saito T, Shimazaki Y. Metabolic disorders related to obesity and periodontal disease. Periodontol 2000 2007;43:254–66.
3. Baeza M, Morales A, Cisterna C, et al. Effect of periodontal treatment in patients with periodontitis and diabetes: systematic review and meta-analysis. J Appl Oral Sci 2020;28:e20190248.
4. Dayo AF, Miles DA, Hamann BR. Detection of medial arterial calcification on CBCT images of a patient with undiagnosed type 2 diabetes mellitus: a case report. Gen Dent 2021;69(5):57–61.
5. Munhoz L, Morita L, Nagai AY, et al. Mandibular cortical index in the screening of postmenopausal at low mineral density risk: a systematic review. Dentomaxillofac Radiol 2021;50(4):20200514.
6. Taguchi A, Tanaka R, Kakimoto N, et al. Clinical guidelines for the application of panoramic radiographs in screening for osteoporosis. Oral Radiol 2021;37(2):189–208.
7. Kunzler A, Farmand M. Typical changes in the viscerocranium in acromegaly. J Cranio-Maxillo-Fac Surg 1991;19(8):332–40.
8. Khodarahmi I, Alizai H, Chalian M, et al. Imaging Spectrum of Calvarial Abnormalities. Radiographics 2021;41(4):1144–63.
9. Kawala B, Matthews-Brzozowska T, Bieniasz J, et al. [Dental and skeletal age in children with growth hormone deficiency treated with growth hormone–preliminary report]. Pediatr Endocrinol Diabetes Metab 2007;13(4):210–2.
10. Kelly A, Pomarico L, de Souza IP. Cessation of dental development in a child with idiopathic hypoparathyroidism: a 5-year follow-up. Oral Surg Oral Med Oral Pathol Oral Radiol Endod 2009;107(5):673–7.
11. Priyanthan T, Hermann AP, Bojsen JA, et al. Multiple Focal Brown Tumors (Osteitis Fibrosa Cystica) in a Renal Transplant Recipient. Case Rep Nephrol 2022;2022: 4675041.

12. Sallies M, Titinchi F, Morkel J. Osteopetrosis complicated by osteomyelitis of the maxilla: A rare case report and review of the literature. Dent Med Probl 2020; 57(3):327–32.

13. Athanasiadou E, Vlachou C, Theocharidou A, et al. When a pedodontic examination leads to the diagnosis of osteopetrosis: A case report. Spec Care Dentist 2020;40(1):113–20.

14. Amaya N, Itoiz ME, Paparella ML. Paget's disease of the jaws: Histopathological features of a series of 31 cases. Acta Odontol Latinoam 2021;34(3):257–62.

15. Werner de Castro GR, Heiden GI, Zimmermann AF, et al. Paget's disease of bone: analysis of 134 cases from an island in Southern Brazil: another cluster of Paget's disease of bone in South America. Rheumatol Int 2012;32(3):627–31.

16. Andreu-Arasa VC, Chapman MN, Kuno H, et al. Craniofacial Manifestations of Systemic Disorders: CT and MR Imaging Findings and Imaging Approach. Radiographics 2018;38(3):890–911.

17. Ko E, Akintoye SO, Mupparapu M, et al. Radiographic Diagnosis of Systemic Diseases Manifested in Jaws. Dent Clin 2021;65(3):579–604.

18. Badki SD, Lohe V, Bhowate R, et al. Conventional Radiology in Deep Seated Facial Hemangioma: A Case Report. Cureus 2023;15(2):e35186.

19. Lee A, Patel NA. Systematic review of pediatric mandibular arteriovenous malformations. Int J Pediatr Otorhinolaryngol 2021;150:110942.

20. Gorlin RJ, Goltz RW. Multiple nevoid basal-cell epithelioma, jaw cysts and bifid rib. A syndrome. N Engl J Med 1960;262:908–12.

21. Suzuki M, Nagao K, Hatsuse H, et al. Molecular pathogenesis of keratocystic odontogenic tumors developing in nevoid basal cell carcinoma syndrome. Oral Surg Oral Med Oral Pathol Oral Radiol 2013;116(3):348–53.

22. Bree AF, Shah MR, Group BC. Consensus statement from the first international colloquium on basal cell nevus syndrome (BCNS). Am J Med Genet 2011; 155A(9):2091–7.

23. Bodmer WF, Bailey CJ, Bodmer J, et al. Localization of the gene for familial adenomatous polyposis on chromosome 5. Nature 1987;328(6131):614–6.

24. Wijn MA, Keller JJ, Giardiello FM, et al. Oral and maxillofacial manifestations of familial adenomatous polyposis. Oral Dis 2007;13(4):360–5.

25. Gardner EJ, Richards RC. Multiple cutaneous and subcutaneous lesions occurring simultaneously with hereditary polyposis and osteomatosis. Am J Hum Genet 1953;5(2):139–47.

26. Cruz-Correa M, Giardiello FM. Familial adenomatous polyposis. Gastrointest Endosc 2003;58(6):885–94.

27. Seehra J, Patel S, Bryant C. Gardner's Syndrome revisited: a clinical case and overview of the literature. J Orthod 2016;43(1):59–64.

28. Kubo K, Miyatani H, Takenoshita Y, et al. Widespread radiopacity of jaw bones in familial adenomatosis coli. J Cranio-Maxillo-Fac Surg 1989;17(8):350–3.

29. Takeuchi T, Takenoshita Y, Kubo K, et al. Natural course of jaw lesions in patients with familial adenomatosis coli (Gardner's syndrome). Int J Oral Maxillofac Surg 1993;22(4):226–30.

30. Mundlos S. Cleidocranial dysplasia: clinical and molecular genetics. J Med Genet 1999;36(3):177–82.

31. Thaweesapphithak S, Saengsin J, Kamolvisit W, et al. Cleidocranial dysplasia and novel RUNX2 variants: dental, craniofacial, and osseous manifestations. J Appl Oral Sci 2022;30:e20220028.

32. Pinheiro M, Freire-Maia N. Ectodermal dysplasias: a clinical classification and a causal review. Am J Med Genet 1994;53(2):153–62.

33. Crawford PJ, Aldred MJ, Clarke A. Clinical and radiographic dental findings in X linked hypohidrotic ectodermal dysplasia. J Med Genet 1991;28(3):181–5.

34. Dogan MS, Callea M, Yavuz I, et al. An evaluation of clinical, radiological and three-dimensional dental tomography findings in ectodermal dysplasia cases. Med Oral Patol Oral Cir Bucal 2015;20(3):e340–6.

35. Lexner MO, Bardow A, Hertz JM, et al. Anomalies of tooth formation in hypohidrotic ectodermal dysplasia. Int J Paediatr Dent 2007;17(1):10–8.

36. Bergendal B. Orodental manifestations in ectodermal dysplasia-a review. Am J Med Genet 2014;164A(10):2465–71.

37. MacDonald-Jankowski D. Fibrous dysplasia: a systematic review. Dentomaxillofac Radiol 2009;38(4):196–215.

38. Hartley I, Zhadina M, Collins MT, et al. Fibrous Dysplasia of Bone and McCune-Albright Syndrome: A Bench to Bedside Review. Calcif Tissue Int 2019;104(5):517–29.

39. Vescini F, Falchetti A, Tonelli V, et al. Mazabraud's Syndrome: A Case Report and Up-To-Date Literature Review. Endocr, Metab Immune Disord: Drug Targets 2019;19(6):885–93.

40. Mainville GN, Turgeon DP, Kauzman A. Diagnosis and management of benign fibro-osseous lesions of the jaws: a current review for the dental clinician. Oral Dis 2017;23(4):440–50.

41. Burke AB, Collins MT, Boyce AM. Fibrous dysplasia of bone: craniofacial and dental implications. Oral Dis 2017;23(6):697–708.

42. de Leval L, Jaffe ES. Lymphoma Classification. Cancer J 2020;26(3):176–85.

43. Triantafillidou K, Dimitrakopoulos J, Iordanidis F, et al. Extranodal non-hodgkin lymphomas of the oral cavity and maxillofacial region: a clinical study of 58 cases and review of the literature. J Oral Maxillofac Surg 2012;70(12):2776–85.

44. Kwok HM, Ng FH, Chau CM, et al. Multimodality imaging of extra-nodal lymphoma in the head and neck. Clin Radiol 2022;77(8):e549–59.

45. de Arruda JAA, Schuch LF, Conte Neto N, et al. Oral and oropharyngeal lymphomas: A multi-institutional collaborative study. J Oral Pathol Med 2021;50(6):603–12.

46. Ardekian L, Rachmiel A, Rosen D, et al. Burkitt's lymphoma of the oral cavity in Israel. J Cranio-Maxillo-Fac Surg 1999;27(5):294–7.

47. Gomes NR, Lima LA, Morais-Perdigao AL, et al. Radiological aspects of lymphomas and leukaemias affecting the jaws: A systematic review. J Oral Pathol Med 2023;52(4):315–23.

48. de Sena A, de Arruda JAA, Costa FPD, et al. Leukaemic infiltration in the oral and maxillofacial region: An update. J Oral Pathol Med 2021;50(6):558–64.

49. Hou GL, Huang JS, Tsai CC. Analysis of oral manifestations of leukemia: a retrospective study. Oral Dis 1997;3(1):31–8.

50. de Sena A, de Arruda JAA, Bemquerer LM, et al. Leukemia/lymphoma oral infiltration and its impact on disease outcomes: A Brazilian study. Oral Dis 2022;29(7):2944–53.

51. Tseng CH, Wang WC, Chen CY, et al. Clinical manifestations of oral lymphomas - Retrospective study of 15 cases in a Taiwanese population and a review of 592 cases from the literature. J Formos Med Assoc 2021;120(1 Pt 2):361–70.

52. Silva TD, Ferreira CB, Leite GB, et al. Oral manifestations of lymphoma: a systematic review. Ecancermedicalscience 2016;10:665.

53. MacDonald D, Martin M, Savage K. Maxillofacial lymphomas. Br J Radiol 2021;94(1120):20191041.

54. Kemp S, Gallagher G, Kabani S, et al. Oral non-Hodgkin's lymphoma: review of the literature and World Health Organization classification with reference to 40 cases. Oral Surg Oral Med Oral Pathol Oral Radiol Endod 2008;105(2):194–201.

55. Buchanan A, Kalathingal S, Capes J, et al. Unusual presentation of extranodal diffuse large B-cell lymphoma in the head and neck: description of a case with emphasis on radiographic features and review of the literature. Dentomaxillofac Radiol 2015;44(3):20140288.

56. Rocha TG, Feitosa EF, Maiolino A, et al. Imaginological characterization of multiple myeloma lesions of the jaws through cone-beam computed tomography. Oral Radiol 2020;36(2):168–76.

57. Cardoso RC, Gerngross PJ, Hofstede TM, et al. The multiple oral presentations of multiple myeloma. Support Care Cancer 2014;22(1):259–67.

58. Kazandjian D. Multiple myeloma epidemiology and survival: A unique malignancy. Semin Oncol 2016;43(6):676–81.

59. Stanborough RO, Garner HW. Multiple myeloma: a review of atypical imaging features and other distinct plasma cell disorders that demonstrate similar imaging features. Skeletal Radiol 2022;51(1):135–44.

60. Bird SA, Boyd K. Multiple myeloma: an overview of management. Palliat Care Soc Pract 2019;13. 1178224219868235.

61. Ormond Filho AG, Carneiro BC, Pastore D, et al. Whole-Body Imaging of Multiple Myeloma: Diagnostic Criteria. Radiographics 2019;39(4):1077–97.

62. Epstein JB, Voss NJ, Stevenson-Moore P. Maxillofacial manifestations of multiple myeloma. An unusual case and review of the literature. Oral Surg Oral Med Oral Pathol 1984;57(3):267–71.

63. Rajkumar SV, Kumar S. Multiple Myeloma: Diagnosis and Treatment. Mayo Clin Proc 2016;91(1):101–19.

64. Furutani M, Ohnishi M, Tanaka Y. Mandibular involvement in patients with multiple myeloma. J Oral Maxillofac Surg 1994;52(1):23–5.

65. Zamagni E, Cavo M. The role of imaging techniques in the management of multiple myeloma. Br J Haematol 2012;159(5):499–513.

66. Rajkumar SV, Dimopoulos MA, Palumbo A, et al. International Myeloma Working Group updated criteria for the diagnosis of multiple myeloma. Lancet Oncol 2014;15(12):e538–48.

67. Kanellias N, Ntanasis-Stathopoulos I, Gavriatopoulou M, et al. Newly Diagnosed Multiple Myeloma Patients with Skeletal-Related Events and Abnormal MRI Pattern Have Poor Survival Outcomes: A Prospective Study on 370 Patients. J Clin Med 2022;11(11):3088.

68. Zamagni E, Tacchetti P, Cavo M. Imaging in multiple myeloma: How? When? Blood 2019;133(7):644–51.

69. Angtuaco EJ, Fassas AB, Walker R, et al. Multiple myeloma: clinical review and diagnostic imaging. Radiology 2004;231(1):11–23.

70. Hirshberg A, Berger R, Allon I, et al. Metastatic tumors to the jaws and mouth. Head Neck Pathol 2014;8(4):463–74.

71. Servato JP, de Paulo LF, de Faria PR, et al. Metastatic tumours to the head and neck: retrospective analysis from a Brazilian tertiary referral centre. Int J Oral Maxillofac Surg 2013;42(11):1391–6.

72. Lopes AM, Freitas F, Vilares M, et al. Metastasis of malignant tumors to the oral cavity: Systematic review of case reports and case series. J Stomatol Oral Maxillofac Surg 2023;124(1S):101330.

73. Irani S. Metastasis to the Jawbones: A review of 453 cases. J Int Soc Prev Community Dent 2017;7(2):71–81.

74. Shintaku WH, Venturin JS, Yepes JF. Application of advanced imaging modalities for the diagnosis of metastatic adenocarcinoma of the lungs in the temporomandibular joint. Oral Surg Oral Med Oral Pathol Oral Radiol Endod 2009;107(6): e37–41.

75. Shimono H, Hirai H, Oikawa Y, et al. Metastatic tumors in the oral region: a retrospective chart review of clinical characteristics and prognosis. Oral Surg Oral Med Oral Pathol Oral Radiol 2021;132(6):648–52.

76. Hirshberg A, Leibovich P, Buchner A. Metastatic tumors to the jawbones: analysis of 390 cases. J Oral Pathol Med 1994;23(8):337–41.

77. de Carvalho Kimura T, FAN Henschel, Carneiro MC, et al. Oral metastasis as the first indication of undiscovered malignancy at a distant site: A systematic review of 413 cases. Head Neck 2022;44(7):1715–24.

78. Kirschnick LB, Schuch LF, Cademartori MG, et al. Metastasis to the oral and maxillofacial region: A systematic review. Oral Dis 2022;28(1):23–32.

79. Hirshberg A, Shnaiderman-Shapiro A, Kaplan I, et al. Metastatic tumours to the oral cavity - pathogenesis and analysis of 673 cases. Oral Oncol 2008;44(8): 743–52.

Moving?

Make sure your subscription moves with you!

To notify us of your new address, find your **Clinics Account Number** (located on your mailing label above your name), and contact customer service at:

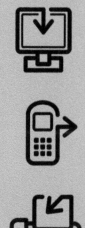

Email: journalscustomerservice-usa@elsevier.com

800-654-2452 (subscribers in the U.S. & Canada)
314-447-8871 (subscribers outside of the U.S. & Canada)

Fax number: 314-447-8029

Elsevier Health Sciences Division
Subscription Customer Service
3251 Riverport Lane
Maryland Heights, MO 63043

Printed and bound by CPI Group (UK) Ltd, Croydon, CR0 4YY

03/10/2024

01040476-0003